I0049974

Lecture Notes in
Medical Diagnosis and Treatment

Immunotherapeutic Approaches for Neurological Diseases:
Natural Monoclonal Antibodies and Conventional Monoclonal Antibodies

Lecture Notes in
Medical Diagnosis and Treatment

Immunotherapeutic Approaches for Neurological Diseases: Natural Monoclonal Antibodies and Conventional Monoclonal Antibodies

Jens O. Watzlawik

Bharath Wootla

Moses Rodriguez

Published by iConcept Press Limited

Published by iConcept Press Limited

Copyright © iConcept Press 2016

http://www.iconceptpress.com

ISBN: 978-1-922227-393

Printed in the United States of America

This work is subjected to copyright.

All rights are reserved, whether the whole or part of the materials is concerned, specifically the rights of translation, reprinting, re-use of illustrations, recitation, broadcasting, reproduction on microfilms or in other ways, and storage in data banks. Duplication of this publication or parts thereof is only permitted under the provisions of the authors, editors and/or iConcept Press Limited.

Contents

Preface

Immunoglobulins with germline sequences occur in invertebrates and vertebrates and are named 'natural antibodies' (NAbs). NAbs are generated in newborns in the absence of external stimulation. They may target foreign antigens, self- or altered self-components and are part of the normal immunoglobulin repertoire. NAbs can act as systemic surveillance molecules, which tag damaged or stressed cells, invading pathogens and toxic protein aggregates for elimination by the immune system. In addition to acting as detecting molecules, certain NAbs actively signal in different cell types with a broad range of responses from induction of apoptosis in cancer cells, stimulation of remyelination in glial cells and blocking disease propagation in neurodegenerative disorders. This lecture note emphasizes the different functions and characteristics of NAbs and their use as potential therapeutics in multiple sclerosis (MS) as an example for neuroinflammatory diseases. Within neurodegenerative diseases we will focus on Alzheimer's disease as the best investigated disease for immunotherapeutic approaches. We will emphasize conventional antibodies and NAbs as a potential future alternative for the treatment of neurodegenerative diseases. In addition, we will highlight the role of the blood brain barrier (BBB) as the major obstacle for antibody based therapies of CNS diseases and stress on some novel approaches to lower the hurdle.

Acknowledgements

This work was supported by grants from the NIH (R01 GM092993, R01 NS048357 and R21 NS073684) and the National Multiple Sclerosis Society (CA 1060A). This work was also supported by a High-Impact Pilot and

Feasibility Award (HIPFA) and Novel Methodology Award (NMDA) from the Mayo Clinic Center for Translational Science Activities (CTSA) and Mayo Clinic CTSA grant number UL1 TR000135 from the National Center for Advancing Translational Science (NCATS), a component of the National Institutes of Health (NIH). We also acknowledge with thanks support from the Applebaum, Hilton, Peterson and Sanford Foundations, the Minnesota Partnership Award for Biotechnology and Medical Genomics and the McNeilus family.

Jens O. Watzlawik
Departments of Neurology and Immunology
Mayo Clinic College of Medicine
Rochester, Minnesota, USA

Bharath Wootla
Departments of Neurology and Immunology
Mayo Clinic College of Medicine
Rochester, Minnesota, USA

Moses Rodriguez
Departments of Neurology and Immunology
Mayo Clinic College of Medicine
Rochester, Minnesota, USA

1

Introduction

Immunoglobulins with germline sequences occur in invertebrates and vertebrates and are named 'natural antibodies' (NAbs). NAbs are generated in newborns in the absence of external stimulation (1). They may target foreign antigens, self- or altered self-components and are part of the normal immunoglobulin repertoire. NAbs act as systemic surveillance molecules, which tag damaged or stressed cells, invading pathogens and toxic protein aggregates for elimination by the immune system. In addition to acting as detecting molecules, certain NAbs actively signal in different cell types with a broad range of responses from induction of apoptosis in cancer cells, stimulation of remyelination in glial cells and blocking disease propagation in neurodegenerative disorders. This lecture note emphasizes the different functions and characteristics of NAbs and conventional antibodies and their use as potential therapeutics in multiple sclerosis (MS) as an example for neuroinflammatory diseases. Within neurodegenerative diseases we will focus on Alzheimer's disease (AD) as the best investigated disease for immunotherapeutic approaches. We will highlight some conventional antibodies and NAbs as potential therapeutics for the treatment of AD and discuss recent failures in clinical trials. In addition, we will emphasize the role of the blood brain barrier (BBB) as the major obstacle for antibody based therapies of CNS diseases and stress on some novel approaches to lower the hurdle.

1.1   Natural Antibodies

Even though the existence of NAbs (also sometimes termed "naturally occurring antibodies") was met with initial skepticism, pioneering work by

Avrameas (2–4) and Notkins (5–8), established convincing evidence that NAbs are part of the human innate immunoglobulin repertoire (3, 9).

NAbs utilize germline-encoded genes directed against foreign antigens, self- and altered self-structures (2) and are present in newborns without stimulation by foreign antigens (10). In contrast, conventional antibodies require external stimuli for their production. NAbs are polyreactive by definition with few or no somatic mutations in the antibody's variable light and heavy chain, which are required for high affinity binding of a single antigen. NAbs of the IgM isotype are found in invertebrates and vertebrates. High levels of IgG NAbs and to a lower extent IgM and IgA isotypes are detected in vertebrates (11). In general, NAbs bind their antigen with low affinity but high avidity (12), which describes the combined synergistic strength of multiple bond interactions rather than the sum of bonds between antigen and antibody. In contrast, conventional antibodies, typically of the IgG isotype, undergo affinity maturation and contain somatic mutations to ensure high-affinity antigen binding, which is commonly linked to the antibody's monospecificity.

Accumulating evidence categorize NAbs as natural systemic surveillance molecules that tag damaged cells and foreign pathogens for elimination by the immune system through opsonization or antibody-dependent cellular cytotoxicity. Some NAbs can actively signal in cancer and brain cells. The ability of identified NAbs to detect and sometimes induce apoptosis in tumor cells may play an important function in tumor surveillance (13–16). In mice and humans, another class of NAbs, termed remyelination promoting antibodies, actively promotes repair in demyelinated spinal cord areas (17–19).

1.2   NAbs-Producing B-cells

Early studies by *Hooijkaas et al.* (1985) and *Van Oudenaren et al.*, (1984) in Specific Pathogen-Free (SPF) mice demonstrated the antigen-independent development of spontaneous IgM-secreting cells in spleen and bone marrow (20, 21). The phenotype of these cells was undetermined and it was also unclear what regulates the induction and maintenance of natural antibody producing cells. Another important question to be addressed was whether natural antibody producing cells follow a similar B cell differentiation pathway compared to B cells induced by foreign antigen challenge.

Animal studies were able to distinguish the B-1 cell subset (previously known as Ly-1 B cells, or CD5+ B cells) and their secreting antibodies from conventional B-2 cells and Marginal zone B cells through allotype-specific markers and demonstrated that B-1 cells are the major natural antibody-producing B cell population in the circulation, in intestinal mucosal tissue and in the respiratory tract (22–25). Antibodies produced by B-1 cells are most often of the IgM isotype followed by IgG and IgA (26, 27). B-1 cells are rare in secondary lymphoid tissues such as lymph nodes and spleen and have not been reported to exist in the bone marrow. Instead they are the major B cell population in peritoneal and pleural cavities (for review see (28)). Ever since the discovery of B-1 cells in these cavities, natural IgM secretion has been attributed to those sites (29–31). It is still under debate whether B-1 cells in peritoneal and pleural cavities are spontaneously able to produce natural IgM antibodies or whether internal or external trigger (e.g. cytokines, LPS) are required to cause B-1 cell migration into the spleen with subsequent differentiation into IgM secreting cells (32–35). In contrast to mature follicular B cells (B2 cells), which typically mediate T-cell responses, mature B-1 cells mediate innate immune responses most likely towards carbohydrate and lipid antigens.

Murine B-1 clones are self-regenerating to ensure the maintenance of this cellular repertoire. During aging the capacity of mature B-1 cells for self-replication becomes limited. To properly phenotype B-1 cells, in addition to CD5, *Rothstein et al.*, has reported a detailed phenotyping scheme for identifying human B-1 cells. Currently, B-1 cells are usually identified by a combination of at least six cell surface markers, having the phenotype CD19^{hi}CD23$^-$CD43$^+$IgM^{hi}IgD$^{(variable)}$CD5$^{\pm}$ (28). The repertoire of these human B-1 cells also appeared to include prominent expression of self-specificities for native DNA and PC-containing antigens (36).

1.3   Polyreactive NAbs

The existence of polyreactive monoclonal antibodies was refuted initially due to the immunological paradigm that antibodies engage antigens with high-affinity in a monospecific manner (37). Ever since, antibodies are expected to target their antigen with high affinity and in a (mono-) specific manner. Polyreactive antibodies with germline origin are mostly ineffective as detecting agents in cell biological or biochemical settings where promiscuous binding of antibodies is commonly equalized with "non-specific binding".

The establishment of natural antibody occurrence in physiological conditions by Avrameas (2–4) and Notkins (5–8) led to greater acceptance of the polyreactivity concept of antibodies. Antibodies are polyreactive when they sufficiently detect more than one antigen (self or foreign). Adequate proof of monospecificity, on the other hand, is commonly accepted in arrays with $> 10^4$ antigens. In the past, antibody monospecificity was not tested to this extent. More recently, when six commercially available monoclonal and polyclonal antibodies were tested on high-density protein arrays comprising of ~ 10,000 recombinant human proteins (Imagenes), four of the antibodies, anti-HSP90, anti-HSA, anti-bFGF and anti-Ro52, showed strong cross-reactivity with other proteins on the array (38). It is unclear to what extent previously classified monospecific antibodies would pass the present criteria in antigen arrays of higher than 10^4 antigens.

Polyreactivity of a single immunoglobulin was formally proven in monoclonal antibodies produced by i) hybridoma technology; ii) Epstein-Barr transfected B lymphocytes; and iii) from patients with B-cell malignancies (39) with polyreactive antibodies from all isotypes (40). Polyreactivity of antibodies is highly conserved in evolution and can even be found in sharks (41). The affinity of polyreactive NAbs to their different antigens can vary by a factor 1000 and is, in general, lower ($K_d = 10^{-3}$ to 10^{-7} mol/L) compared to affinity-maturated monospecific antibodies (conventional antibodies) ($K_d = 10^{-7}$ to 10^{-11} mol/L) (42) (Table 1).

The half-life of polyreactive natural antibodies *in vivo* is significantly shorter compared to monospecific ones (Table 1). The rapid serum clearance of polyreactive monoclonal antibodies is likely due to binding to multiple endogenous antigens.

1.3.1   Antigen Binding Mechanism of Polyspecific Natural Antibodies

Transferring the CDR3 region of the heavy Ig chain from a polyreactive to a monospecific antibody induces polyreactivity (43). Supporting evidence comes from studies demonstrating that isolated amino-acid replacements within the CDRH3 region of polyreactive antibodies are sufficient to create monospecific antibodies (44, 45). Thus far, no differences in the conformation, amino acid chain length or sequence can be detected in the CDRH3 regions of monospecific versus polyreactive antibodies (42). In addition, a single amino-acid replacement outside the antigen-binding pocket is sufficient to abolish polyreactivity (39). Thus, not only the antibodies paratope but also the whole variable domain is essential for polyreactivity.

	Polyreactive Monoclonal Antibody	Monospecific Monoclonal Antibody
Antigen	Many structurally diverse and unrelated antigens	Single antigen
Affinity	Low (K_d: 10^{-4} to 10^{-7})	High (K_d: 10^{-7} to 10^{-11})
Sequence	Germline or near germline with few somatic mutations, no affinity maturation	Somatically mutated, affinity maturated
Number of potentially allowed conformations inside the antibody's antigen binding pocket	More than one conformation allowed	Only one conformation allowed (lock and key fit mechanism)
Immunoglobulin subtype	IgM > IgA and IgG	IgG > IgM, IgA
Half-life time	IgM:~8 h; IgG: ~10 h; IgA: ~8 h	IgM:~35 h; IgG: ~280 h; IgA: ~26 h

Table 1: Properties of polyreactive versus monospecific monoclonal antibodies

There is a higher degree of glycosylation on polyreactive monoclonal antibodies relative to monospecific monoclonal antibodies (46). Bulky carbohydrate moieties attached to the variable regions of immunoglobulins contribute to protein conformation (47). Glycosylation of the immunoglobulin's variable domain can interfere with its ability to target its antigen (48); this may be an alternative explanation for a higher degree of variability in the antigen-antibody interaction as seen with polyreactive antibodies compared with monoreactive antibodies.

Several mechanistic theories have been proposed to explain polyspecificity (42). Of those, the **induced fit** hypothesis and the **conformational selection** theory are explained here in more detail (Figure 1): The induced fit theory proposes a flexible antibody paratope capable of undergoing multiple favorable conformations, which are induced and stabilized by the approaching antigen L (Figure 1, right side). The antigen L shifts the equilibrium between the two proposed conformations towards conformation 3 (Figure 1, right side). The different arrow types between both conformations indicates the shift in the equilibrium between conformations 3 and 4 upon antigen approach.

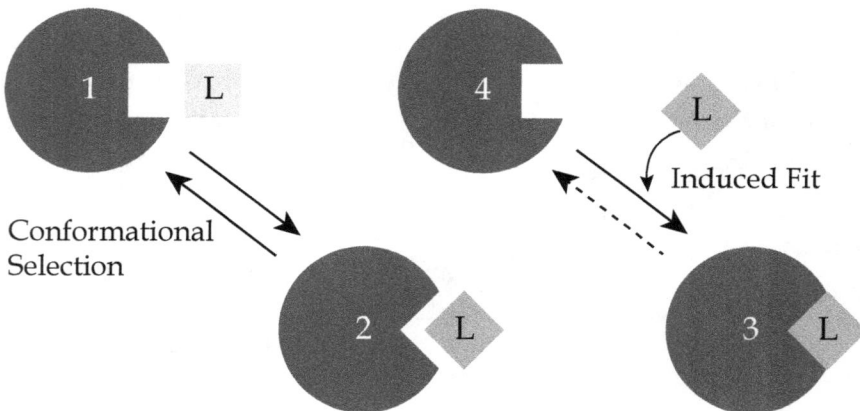

Figure 1: Explanation of polyspecificity by using induced fit hypothesis and conformational selection theory. On the right: induced fit theory. On the left: conformational selection theory.

The induced fit theory is thermodynamically reasonable, but kinetically likely too slow to have a significant impact for antigen-antibody recognition. This is, because formation of the energetically unstable initial antigen-antibody complex is rate-limiting (49). Supporting data for the induced fit theory comes from a study showing conformational changes in a germ-line encoded polyreactive antibody (Fab-fragment) compared to its affinity matured isoform upon hapten-binding (50). The paratope conformation of the germ-line antibody changed upon binding to the hapten, whereas the affinity matured antibody targets the hapten by a **lock and key fit mechanism** without major conformational changes within the protein-binding site (50).

The **conformational selection** theory on the other hand proposes similarly to the induced fit theory a flexible paratope with, however, pre-existing multiple conformations (Figure 1, left side). The approaching antigens L (blue and green) have no impact on the equilibrium between conformations 1 and 2 (equally long arrows between conformational stages 1 and 2 in Figure 1). In addition, the different paratope conformations may be stabilized through interactions with regions outside the paratope or environmental factors (solvent, temperature, pH) (51). Compared with the former model the conformational selection theory ensures significantly higher reaction rates. In addition, growing experimental evidence supports the conformational selection theory (49).

Alternative explanations for polyspecificity are i) **flexible antigens:** a set of flexible antigens could bind to the same antibody (52). Carbohydrate ligands present on glycoproteins and glycosphingolipids as well as small peptide ligands are intrinsically flexible and different carbohydrate epitopes or peptides could cross-react even with a single rigid antibody paratope, ii) **public epitopes:** public epitopes are often found on carbohydrates, where different carbohydrates interact similarly through different hydrogen-bonds with key atoms inside the antibody binding-site (53). iii) **large paratopes:** structural analysis demonstrated that protein epitopes (antigen) are commonly limited to three to seven amino acids (54). The antibody's paratope is, however, often larger in size than the antigen's epitope. Therefore, different antigens could interact with different regions of the paratope through entirely different interactions.

Polyreactivity *in vitro*

Polyreactivity seen in purified antibodies may, however, not always be an intrinsic property of the immunoglobulin, but instead induced by physico-chemical treatments under *in vitro* and *in vivo* conditions. Antibody polyreactivity *in vitro* can be induced by denaturing agents/conditions (chaotropic agents, pH, temperature) during the antibody purification process. Alternatively, polyreactivity may be the result of immunoglobulin expression in hybridoma cell lines with different glycosylation patterns compared to the serum derived natural antibody, which, in addition, varies from cell line to cell line (55).

Polyreactivity *in vivo*

Induction of antibody polyspecificity may also occur *in vivo*. In ischemia-reperfusion injury, an inappropriate activation of the complement system mediates a severe inflammatory response resulting in tissue damage. This process is initiated by natural antibodies (56). Macromolecules such as antibodies are easily oxidized under inflammatory conditions by reactive oxygen species (ROS) as demonstrated *in vivo* (57). Close contact of antibodies with ROS-producing activated neutrophils results in an enhancement of bacterial antigen recognition through induction or increase of polyreactivity (58). It has been proven that some antibodies acquire polyspecificity after circulating through inflammation sites (59). This effect may enhance the innate immune systems capacity to act as or strengthen the first line of defense, where certain immunoglobulins are not only targets of ROS but capable to facilitate their own generation (60).

1.4   Common Antigens and Function of Autoreactive Natural Antibodies

Pathogenic self-reactive antibodies are sorted out at several checkpoints during lymphocyte differentiation to prevent autoimmune diseases. However, certain autoreactive immune cells and antibodies are not associated with pathogenesis but potentially play important roles in tissue homeostasis (61) and tumor surveillance (62).

Tissue Homeostasis

Tissue homeostasis is an essential criterion for healthy populations of cells and entire organs with countless newly generated cells on one side and dying, apoptotic cells on the other side.

A substantial proportion of NAbs with identified antigens target "neo-self" proteins and lipids, which are exposed at the level of the plasma membrane on apoptotic but not on healthy cells (63). Two types of epitopes were identified in human and rodents to dominate the response to apoptotic cells, phosphorylcholine and malondialdehyde (MDA).

Phosphorylcholine is part of the surface exposed, hydrophilic head group of phospholipids. It is also part of the sphingolipid sphingomyelin and the protein platelet-activating factor (PAF). All these molecules are ubiquitous cellular components respective present in many different cell types. One of the best characterized B-1 cell clones, T15, produces IgMs, which target phosphorylcholine on apoptotic cells, oxidized LDL as well as phosphorylcholine covalently linked to a bacterial cell wall (64).

Malondialdehyde (MDA) is an aldehyde-containing degradation product from unsaturated lipids through contact with reactive oxidation species (65). MDA is assayed *in vivo* as a biomarker of oxidative stress (66) and forms covalent protein and mutagenic DNA adducts (67). These two epitopes (MDA or phosphorylcholine) represent about 50 % of all epitopes on apoptotic cells detected by IgMs (65). Other apoptosis-associated antigens detected by natural IgM antibodies are cardiolipin, annexin IV and phosphatidylserine (PS) (68).

Antibodies targeting apoptotic cells may have therapeutic potential in various diseases with lost control of apoptosis (e.g. neurodegenerative diseases, immune compromised patients). In general, cell death is necessary for normal development of cells, tissues and organs. However, the inability of the immune system to clear dead, apoptotic cells compromises development in healthy individuals and under disease states. Accumulation of apoptotic cells under pathogenic conditions may result in exacerbation of the disease. Therefore, natural antibodies targeting apoptotic cells may be beneficial for a variety of diseases.

Other NAbs target cell surface antigens on erythrocytes either exposed during their senescence, or experimentally induced proteolytic damage of red blood cells (69). Instead of undergoing apoptosis red blood cell senescence is associated with a different plasma membrane associated change, which is detectable by natural antibodies.

In summary, humans and mice have at least two different sets of NAbs, which either target senescent erythrocytes or apoptotic cells. Natural antibodies targeting these cells have been postulated to reinforce immune homeostasis (61) and may have therapeutic potential in multiple diseases. NAbs may also be used as detecting agents for tumors with high cellular apoptosis rates.

Tumor Surveillance

Despite decades of extensive cancer research potent and at the same time selective therapeutics targeting tumor cells are rare. Long term prognosis in patients with progressive, metastasized tumors is typically poor. Thus, better therapeutic approaches are needed to combat advanced tumor stages.

Malignant cells often express cell surface proteins with modified glycosylation pattern compared to healthy cells. Modified carbohydrates on glycoproteins and glycolipids can form "neo-self' epitopes, which are detectable by natural antibodies on tumor cells only (70). The nature of these self-repeating carbohydrate epitopes allows multivalent IgM molecules to bind with high avidity to its target (NAbs as tumor detecting agents). This activates the complement cascade to destroy IgM-tagged cancer cells. Unfortunately, cancer cells are protected from complement attack through cell-surface receptors including complement receptor 1, decay accelerating factor (DAF), protectin, and membrane cofactor protein (MCP), which control activation of complement C3 or prevent formation of the membrane attack complex (71, 72). However, efficient IgMs can inhibit factors important for tumor proliferation, survival or metastases. The monoclonal IgM SAM-6 targets an O-linked carbohydrate attached to the heat shock protein GRP78 (15). HSPs are cytoplasmic proteins in healthy cells, but they can be found at the level of the plasma membrane in neoplastic cells (73), where they may act as signaling receptors (74, 75). Endocytic internalization of the IgM SAM-6 results in accumulation of oxidized lipoproteins, which in turn induces apoptosis in tumor cells (NAbs as tumor cell killers) (13, 14).

Numerous human monoclonal antibodies targeting tumor cells were produced by hybridoma technology and derived from human neoplastic cells and human control cells. Interestingly, all identified antibodies were of the IgM isotype (76). Fourteen of the tumor-reactive monoclonal IgMs were selected and analyzed based on their binding characteristics, DNA sequence, their origin and genetics. All selected IgMs were germline encoded and of B1-cell origin, bound to carbohydrate epitopes on tumor specific receptors and induced apoptosis (76). A ring cell carcinoma derived human monoclonal antibody, termed SC-1, induced apoptosis of stomach cancer cells *in vitro* (77) and *in vivo* (78–80). SC-1 targets a modified form of the membrane bound antigen CD55. Clinical studies with SC-1 in cancer patients demonstrated tumor regression and apoptosis of cancer cells with no signs of toxicity towards healthy tissue (81).

Ten year survival rates of patients with CD55-positive gastric cancer receiving a single dose of the antibody before surgery demonstrate a 55 % survival rate in those patients receiving the antibody compared to 30 % survival rate in patients with surgery only (http://www.patrys.net.au/product-pipeline/clinical-products/patrys-pat-sc1). This clearly indicates a beneficial effect of the antibody treatment. It is undetermined whether multiple antibody doses are even more potent in patients with CD55-positive gastric cancer.

There is sufficient proof that a number of IgM NAbs targeting neoepitopes on cancer cells induce apoptosis *in vivo* and *in vitro*. These IgMs are part of the innate immune response and may be responsible for natural defense against tumors in healthy individuals (tumor surveillance). It suggests that the innate or natural immunity, which was defined as rather non-specific response, is more important than initially expected (82).

2

Immunotherapies using Conventional and Natural Antibodies for the Treatment of Multiple Sclerosis (MS)

2.1 Immunosuppressive and Immunomodulatory Therapeutic Approaches for MS

MS is the most common chronic inflammatory, demyelinating disease of the CNS and typically results in neurological disability. Current therapies using glatiramer acetate, β-interferons, immune suppressive agents, or adhesion molecule inhibitors ease the severity of acute attacks and lower their frequency but result in the same degree of long-term disability as seen in placebo treated patients. In addition, strong immune suppressive drugs facilitate fatal infections. We believe a paradigm shift is necessary from immunosuppressive/immunomodulatory strategies in MS, which aim to prevent disease exacerbation, towards active regenerative strategies, which intend to repair demyelinated brain and spinal cord lesions.

Here we discuss different immune therapy options with focus on **monoclonal antibodies** as potential therapeutic strategies for MS patients.

2.1.1 US Food and Drug Administration (FDA)-Approved Monoclonal Antibodies for The Treatment of MS

So far, Natalizumab and Alemtuzumab are the only US Food and Drug Administration (FDA)-approved monoclonal antibody for the treatment of MS.

A. Natalizumab (Tysabri)

Natalizumab is a humanized monoclonal antibody that targets the focal adhesion molecule integrin α-4 present on T lymphocytes and other immune cells. Integrin α-4 is essential for T lymphocytes to cross the BBB and enter the CNS lesion site. Natalizumab is effective in an immune-mediated animal model of MS where it prevents T lymphocytes from entering the CNS lesions and thereby lessening the disease (83). When administered every four weeks in a phase III trial, natalizumab reduced the exacerbation rate by approximately 68% (84). Natalizumab combined with beta-interferon resulted in an additional decrease in disease activity (85). However, Natalizumab poses an increased risk of CNS virus infections leading to progressive multifocal leukoencephaolpathy (PML). As of December 2014 there were 517 cases of natalizumab-associated PML among 132,600 patients (http://bitly.com/nat-pml) (86).

B. Alemtuzumab (Campath-1H)

The monoclonal antibody Alemtuzumab (Campath) targets an antigen (CD52) present on monocytes and lymphocytes and causes systemic suppression of the immune system that can last for up to a year. The primary indication for Alemtuzumab is the treatment of chronic lymphocytic leukemia. A phase III trial in patients with relapsing-remitting MS demonstrated lower relapse rates compared to controls but without having an effect on the degree of disability (87). An earlier phase II trial was terminated due to development of idiopathic thrombocytopenia in three patients (87). Approximately 23 % of patients under alemtuzumab develop autoimmune thyroid disease and may be at risk to develop PML or other potentially fatal opportunistic infections.

    The main safety concerns include autoimmune thyroid problems and idiopathic thrombocytopenic purpura (ITP) for which patients will require monitoring.

2.1.2 Non FDA-Approved Monoclonal Antibodies for the Treatment of MS

C. Rituximab (Rituxan)

The chimeric monoclonal antibody Rituximab binds and destroys B cells through binding to a phosphorylated glycoprotein (CD20). Rituximab was primarily used for diseases characterized by overactive B cells. Based on antibody-mediated injury seen in an immune-mediated animal model of MS (EAE), and its assumed predictive value for relapsing and progressive MS, Rituximab was considered as an alternative treatment for MS and studied in more detail. Rituximab lowers the rate of relapses in MS patients by 50 % as determined 48 weeks after administration (88). However, the clinical outcome in patients with primary progressive disease was not significantly different (89). In addition, Rituximab may also cause PML and is associated with reactivation of dormant prior infections like hepatitis B (90).

D. Daclizumab (Zenepax)

The humanized monoclonal antibody Daclizumab binds to the interleukin-2 receptor (CD25) on T cells, B cells and thymocytes (91). Daclizumab was primarily used to prevent rejection of transplanted organs. With respect to disease related processes CD25 is also expressed in neoplastic B cells, neuroblastomas and tumor infiltrating lymphocytes. Daclizumab improved the MRI outcome and clinical scores in patients with MS in combination with β-interferon or in monotherapy (91). So far, there were no reports of opportunistic infections or other life-threatening adverse effects with daclizumab. This is in contrast to side-effects seen with natalizumab and rituximab and may be based on its rather immune modulatory as opposed to immune suppressive effects. It was assumed that daclizumab eradicates certain CD4 and CD8 T lymphocyte populations through increasing levels of CD56+ natural killer cells (92). A phase III trial using daclizumab versus β-interferon demonstrated a 45 % reduction in annual relapses compared to β-interferon in patients with relapsing multiple sclerosis.

E. Ocrelizumab

The humanized monoclonal antibody Ocrelizumab targets the phosphorylated glycoprotein CD20 (see Rituximab) on circulating B lymphocytes but not plasma cells. Similar to Rituximab, Ocrelizumab causes depletion of B lymphocytes through complement- and antibody-dependent cytotoxicity plus stimulation of apoptosis. An important reason for its development was the detection of anti-chimeric neutralizing antibodies against the chimeric antibody Rituximab in 24 % of patients. This disturbing outcome is likely to be reduced in patients treated with the humanized antibody Oc-relizumab. The favorable outcome in a phase II trial comparing Ocreli-zumab against IFNβ-1a and placebo led to a phase III study in primary progressive MS and relapsing-remitting MS (93). There are, however, safe-ty concerns using Ocrelizumab based on the phase II MS trial noted above with a 41-year old patient dying from brain edema 14 weeks into the trial. A phase III trial of Ocrelizumab in systemic lupus erythematosus was dis-continued due to opportunistic infections after methotrexate exposure (94).

F. Ofatumumab (Arzerra)

Ofatumumab is a fully human monoclonal antibody targeting CD20. Ofatumumab was previously FDA appoved in combination with chlorambucil, for the treatment of previously untreated patients with chronic lymphocytic leukemia (CLL). Results from phase I/II trials using Ofatumumab vs placebo for relapsing-remitting MS reported no major safety concerns. Ofatumumab-treatment resulted in a ≥90% reduction in new T1 gadolinium-enhancing lesions for all doses of Ofatumumab ≥30 mg ($P < 0.001$) (95).

2.1.3 Off-Label use of Polyclonal Intravenous Immunoglobulins (IVIgG) for The Treatment of Relapsing-Remitting Multiple Scle-rosis (RRMS) Patients

Intravenous Immunoglobulins (IVIgG)

IVIgG is a therapeutic compound prepared from pools of plasma obtained from several thousand healthy blood donors. IVIgG contains small amounts of NAbs and typically lacks immunoglobulin isotypes other than IgGs, which is, however, dependent on the manufacturing process used. The advantage of large donor pools is reflected by an increased reactivity of individual antibodies to certain antigens. Theoretically, IVIgG compris-es the entire range of reactivity exhibited by IgG of normal human sera. The reactivity can target foreign antigens, including bacterial and viral an-tigens, as well as self-antigens such as membrane-associated self-molecules, intracellular and extracellular antigens. It was found that the self-reactivity of normal serum IgG with solubilized extracts of normal homologous tissues targeted a conserved and limited set of dominant antigens (96–98). The constant interaction between antibodies, antibody molecules and variable regions of antigen receptors on B cells is an essential component of selection of immune repertoires and establishment of tolerance to self (99, 100).

Components of IVIgG Preparations, Production Process and Product Safety

Intact IgG molecules form the primary component of IVIgG, which is produced by commercial manufacturers as well as not-for-profit organizations. Due to diverse manufacturers in the market, several quality markers of IVIG preparations including purity, pH, osmolarity, sodium and sugar content may vary between IVIgG preparations (101). IVIG preparations undergo viral inactivation and may contain trace amounts of IgA, anti-A and anti-B (IgG antibodies directed against human blood group antigens), soluble CD4, CD8, HLA molecules and certain cytokines (102–104). Most of the methodology used to isolate and purify IVIgG dates back to the late 1950s. The more recently tweaked methodology that includes caprylate precipitation followed by anion exchange chromatography is currently used (105). Characteristics of commercially prepared IVIgG are a pH in the range of 4-6, with ≥240 mosmol/kg, a total protein quantity of ≥30 g/l with ≤3% of immune aggregates. Finally, the product should test negative for the surface antigen of the hepatitis B virus (HBsAg), HIV p24 antigen, anti-HIV-1 antibodies, anti-HIV-2 antibodies and anti-hepatitis C virus (HCV) antibodies (102).

Clinical use of IVIgG Preparations

After demonstrating an attenuated clearance of platelets in a child with immune thrombocytopenic purpura (ITP) (106) followed by a similar effect in adults with ITP (107), IVIgG was licensed for use in ITP. IVIgG was also tested and used in the clinic as a replacement low-dose therapy for primary and secondary immunodeficiencies. Diseases in this category include PID (108), X-linked agammaglobulinaemia (XLA), acquired hypogammaglobulinemia, common variable immunodeficiency, X-linked hyper-immunoglobulin (Ig)M, severe combined immunodeficiency, HIV infection, Wiskott–Aldrich syndrome and selective IgG class deficiency (109, 110). Other currently licensed indications for IVIgG include Kawasaki disease, Guillain-Barrè syndrome, and chronic inflammatory demyelinating polyneuropathy (CIDP). However, its initial success in treatment of ITP led to its use in treating many systemic inflammatory and autoimmune disorders affecting the joints, skin, hematopoietic system and central nervous system (109). Licensed uses account for less than half of the annual worldwide sales of IVIgG preparations; most sales are for "off-label" IVIgG applications (111). In addition to antibody-mediated diseases, IVIgG is also effective in several disorders caused by derailment of cellular immunity, such as dermatomyositis, multiple sclerosis (MS), graft-versus-host disease (GvHD) in recipients of allogeneic bone marrow transplants and treatment of cellular rejection after organ transplantation (112–114).

Mechanisms of action of IVIgG

Infused IVIgG has a half-life of 21 days in immuno-competent individuals; however, the beneficial effect of IVIgG extends beyond its half-life. This suggests that IVIgG therapy not only neutralizes pathogenic antibodies but also induces lasting changes in the cellular compartment of the immune system. The precise mechanism by which IVIgG suppresses inflammation is multi-factorial with many working hypotheses postulated: inhibition of activation of macrophages, dendritic cells, and pathogenic T-cells (Th1 cells, Th17 cells); expansion of regulatory T-cells; modulation of B-cell responses and inhibition of pathogenic autoantibody production; suppression of inflammatory cytokine production; neutralization of pathogenic autoantibodies via anti-idiotypes and inhibition of complement (115).

Potential use of IVIgG for the treatment of relapsing-remitting MS patients

A proven track record of minimal side effects of IVIgG in treated patients and promising data from experimental animal models of MS prompted the initiation of clinical trials for the treatment of relapsing-remitting MS (RRMS).

Initial European clinical studies showed beneficial effects of IVIgG for RRMS. An Austrian study was multicenter, randomized, double-blind and placebo-controlled with patients receiving monthly doses of 0.15–0.2 g/kg for 2 years (116). IVIgG treated patients showed reduced clinical disability levels as measured by the absolute change in Kurtzke's expanded

disability status scale (EDSS) score. The beneficial outcome for RRMS patients was confirmed in 1998 by showing reduced numbers of gadolinium-
enhancing lesions on monthly serial MRI scans in the IVIgG arm of the
study. In addition, the number of exacerbation-free patients was significantly higher during IVIgG treatment. (117). A double-blind, placebo-
controlled study in Poland reported that an IVIgG dose of 0.2 g/kg administered once per month for 12 months is equally effective as 0.4 g/kg in
reducing MS activity (118). Subsequent data from a retrospective, multicenter observational study over 5 years reported that IVIgG treatment
(0.24 ± 0.15 g/kg/month) resulted in 69% reduction in mean annual relapse rate (119). Collectively, these studies suggested that IVIgG is effective in reducing relapse rate in RRMS.

In contrast, a randomized, double-blinded, placebo-controlled trial
of IVIgG immunoglobulin (IVIgG) performed in MS patients with persis-
tent muscle weakness indicated no difference in the degree of change in
strength between treatment groups. There was no apparent benefit in relapse behavior or impairment measures during the 6-month observation
period in 67 enrolled patients. No benefit was observed in either patients
who remained clinically stable or in those with evidence of disease activity. Patients with active MS during the trial worsened in all groups. It was
concluded that IVIgG does not reverse muscle weakness in MS. The iso-
metric muscle strength measurement was a reliable indicator of strength
(120). The negative outcome of IVIgG for the treatment of RRMS was confirmed in the randomized, double-blinded, placebo-controlled PRIVIG
study using two doses of IVIgG or placebo. After 1 year, the differences in
relapse-free patients did not differ statistically between treatment groups
and no difference was observed in numbers of newly active MRI lesions. It
was concluded that IVIgG treatment had no beneficial effect in RRMS
patients in doses ranging from 0.2 to 0.4 g/kg (121). The negative outcome
in both studies seriously questioned the utility of IVIgG for the treatment
of relapsing-remitting multiple sclerosis.

While many autoinflammatory diseases have proved responsive to
IVIgG therapy the outcome of these MS trials is still puzzling. Several
factors may have impacted the different outcome. The heterogeneity of the
disease with likely different underlying pathological mechanisms may
have had a significant impact. Patient cohorts enlisted in trials were not

uniform, relatively small and potentially not comparable between different trials (122).

IVIgG is currently not considered practical for the treatment of MS. IVIgG may prevent relapses after a first demyelinating event, but a beneficial effect in patients with RRMS is unclear. Use of IVIgG may be considered in patients with severe relapses that are non-responsive to corticosteroids (123).

Intravenous IgM, an alternative to Intravenous IgG

Immunoglobulin M (IgM) is an important component discarded during IVIgG preparations. Given the plasma concentration of IgM, ~18 tons of pooled IgM may be discarded every year. Studies performed in the past have documented the beneficial effect of polyclonal human IgM molecules.

Treatment of chronically TMEV-infected mice with polyclonal human IgM resulted in enhanced remyelination when compared with IVIGG. Moreover, polyclonal human IgM promoted remyelination to a degree comparable to the monoclonal human IgM termed rHIgM22 (see 2.2.) (18). IVIgM also prevents complement activation *in vitro* and *in vivo* in a rat model of acute inflammation (124) and inhibits classical pathway complement activation, but not bactericidal activity, of human serum (125). *Stehr et al.*, reported on the use of IgM-enriched solution on polymorphonuclear neutrophil function, bacterial clearance and lung histology in endotoxemia, a condition in which both pro-inflammatory and anti-inflammatory cascade systems are simultaneously initiated similar to sepsis. Their results documented a striking pulmonary protective effect of IVIgM, enhanced reticuloendothelial system bacterial clearance, increased *in vivo* phagocytosis efficiency, and an especially beneficial effect on LPS-induced pulmonary histological changes (126). The *in vivo* therapeutic efficacy of IVIgM was also confirmed in experimental models of uveitis, myasthenia gravis, and multiple sclerosis (17, 18, 127). The mechanisms of action of IVIgM include the induction of apoptosis of lymphoid cell lines and human peripheral blood mononuclear cells (128), the suppression of T cell functions *in vitro* and a delay in the activation of T lymphocytes in SCID mice (129). IVIGgM may overcome, at least in part, the shortage of

IVIgG; however, further work is warranted to appreciate the true beneficial potential of polyclonal IgM antibodies.

2.2   Strategies to Repair CNS Lesions in Multiple Sclerosis Patients using Remyelination Promoting Antibodies (rHIgM22)

Monoclonal remyelination promoting antibodies represent a potential novel class of therapeutics for MS patients with the ability to actively repair CNS lesions in animal models of MS. At the time of this writing, the human monoclonal antibody rHIgM22 successfully completed phase I trial for patients with all clinical presentations of MS (130). In this study, rHIgM22 showed excellent safety and tolerability at all doses tested. Furthermore, HIgM22 was detected in the cerebral spinal fluid (CSF) two days after intravenous injection (i.e., ≥ 0.05 ng/ml) in all rHIgM22-treated patients at two dose levels. Even 29 days after treatment, rHIgM22 was measurable in the CSF of 5 out of 12 patients (131). This human data demonstrates that IgM antibodies are able to cross the BBB and persist in the CSF (> 40 % of patients) for almost a month after treatment.

The remainder of this section emphasizes characteristics of remyelination promoting antibodies, identified antigens and proposed mechanism(s) of action for this antibody class.

2.2.1   Remyelination-Promoting Antibodies are a Subclass of NAbs

All identified monoclonal remyelination promoting antibodies are of germline origin or near germline with few somatic mutations, thus having the cardinal features of physiologic natural antibodies. So far, all identified remyelination promoting antibodies with NAb features are IgMs (O1, O4, A2B5, HNK-1, rHIgM22, except high-affinity anti-Lingo IgG antibodies, which stimulate remyelination in rodents but do not have NAb features).

2.2.2   Characterization of Remyelination-Promoting Antibodies

All remyelination promoting antibodies with known antigens are polyreactive, which is the result of their rather flexible antigen binding site. Thus, antibodies with identified antigens bind to at least one or multiple sphingolipids, which are glycosylated lipids with ceramide or sphingosine backbone and essential lipid raft components. Only the hydrophilic carbohydrate moiety of the sphingolipids is exposed to the cell surface and, therefore, detectable by antibodies. This emphasizes the carbohydrate moiety and excludes the lipid backbone as the essential part of the antigen.

The dissociation constants (K_d) of the monoclonal (mouse) remyelination promoting IgMs O4 and O1 are unusually high for polyreactive natural antibodies ($\sim 0.9 \times 10^{-9}$ M for O4 and O1 compared to K_d's of typically 10^{-4} to 10^{-7} M for natural antibodies) (132) (see also table 1). A study by *Paz Soldan et. al.,* (133) indicated that all tested remyelination promoting IgMs induce a Ca^{2+}-influx in astrocytes (GFAP+), OPCs and immature OLs (133). IgM-mediated effects in astrocytes and oligodendrocytes were, however, independent from each other, based on different signaling mechanisms and based on different Ca^{2+}pools (ER-stored Ca^{2+} for astrocytes and extracellular Ca^{2+} for oligodendrocytes) (133). The AMPA glutamate receptor was shown to be responsible for IgM-mediated calcium-influx into OPCs and immature OLs whereas IgMs-stimulated calcium-influx into astrocytes was mediated through phospholipase C-mediated generation of IP3 and subsequent gating of IP3-sensitive channels (133). In summary, all well-characterized remyelination promoting antibodies are of germline origin, belong to the IgM isotype and induce calcium influx into astrocytes, OPCs and immature OLs.

2.2.3   Common Antigens and Mechanistic Theories for Remyelination Promoting Antibodies

A. Common Antigens

The ganglioside-binding antibody A2B5 targets several sialylated glycosphingolipids (= gangliosides) due to their similar carbohydrate epitope (134). HNK-1 recognizes the glycosphingolipid 3-sulfoglucuronyl paragloboside (SGPG) (135) as well as the carbohydrate epitope of the glycoproteins MAG and P0 (136). The mouse IgM O1 binds to galactocerebroside and similar glycosphingolipids (137), whereas O4 targets sulfated galactocerebroside (sulfatide), seminolipid, the unknown pro-oligodendroblast antigen (POA) and cholesterol (O4) (137).

A more recent study shifted our focus from glycosphingolipids to glycoproteins as an alternative class of antigens for remyelination promoting antibodies. As mentioned earlier, the carbohydrate, but not the lipid moiety of sphingolipids, is accessible to antibodies and may be sufficient for antibody binding when linked to either a lipid or protein backbone. The relatively simple carbohydrate structure on sphingolipids compared to the complex glycosylation found on many glycoproteins suggests that carbohydrate building blocks responsible for antibody binding can be found on glycoproteins as well. *Inoko et al.,* (2010) demonstrated binding of the remyelination promoting IgM A2B5 to a novel set of brain-derived glycoproteins as shown by Western blots (138). It is well accepted that A2B5 binds to c-series gangliosides GT3 and GQ1c. However, c-series gangliosides and their O-acetyl derivatives are majorly expressed during early developmental stages in the CNS but seldom during adulthood in vertebrates (139). Cerebellar stellate neurons are the only known exception in the adult human CNS that express c-series gangliosides (140). This raises the question whether CNS remyelination promotion in adult mice by A2B5 is mediated through binding to glycosphingolipids or glycoproteins (141).

B. Mechanistic Strategies

Glycosphingolipids and cholesterol are essential components of lipid rafts, which act as signaling platforms at the level of the plasma membrane in cells. Lipid rafts may enable or disable interactions between many different cell-surface receptors (proteins) to transduce extracellular stimuli over the plasma membrane into the cytoplasmic space (general lipid raft concept). Pentameric IgM molecules can bind and cluster up to ten antigens at a time on different cells. We hypothesize that IgMs targeting glycosphingolipids stabilize existing rafts or stimulate the formation of new lipid rafts at the plasma membrane, thereby enhancing the effects of extracellular stimuli via existing cellular signaling pathways (**lipid raft hypothesis**).

Alternatively, remyelination-promoting IgMs may be involved in the **opsonization of cellular debris and dead or apoptotic cells** in a lesion site. Remyelination promoting antibodies 94.03 and 79.08 (141), O1 and the human sulfatide binding IgM DS1F8 (142) prominently stain filaments in astrocytes or HeLa cells, which are identified as microtubule-like structures (142). Figure 2 emphasizes binding of remyelination promoting antibodies 94.03 and 79.03 to filamentous structures present in astrocytes (arrows) (Figure 2). Binding to intracellular filamentous structures is also common with antibodies targeting galactosylceramide and sulfatide (143). This may indicate epitope similarities between oligodendrocyte specific

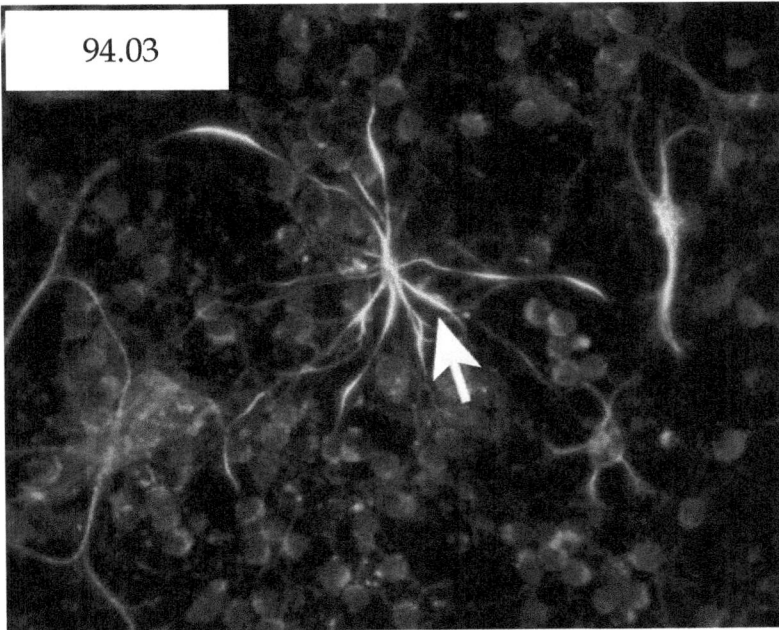

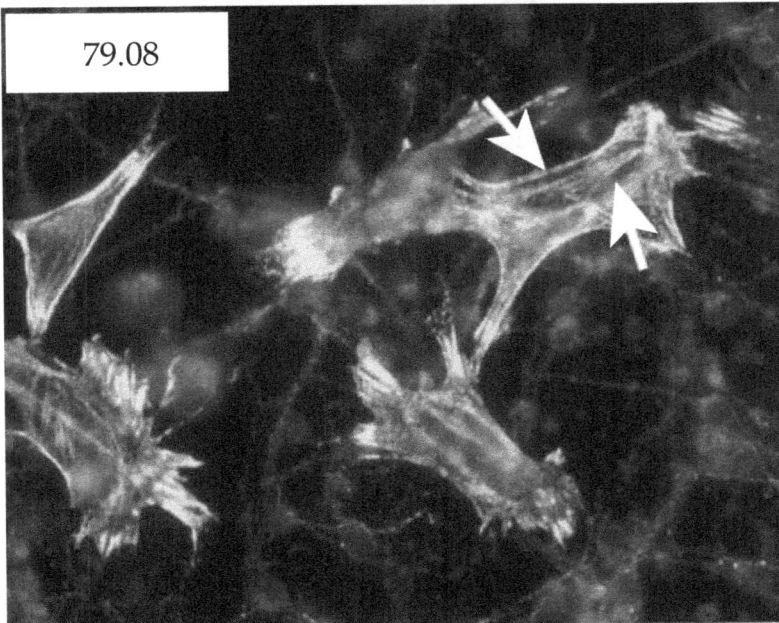

Figure 2: Binding of remyelination promoting antibodies 94.03 and 79.03 to filamentous structures present in astrocytes (arrows).

glycosphingolipids present at the cell surface and in internal pools relative to intracellular cytoskeletal proteins detected by polyreactive antibodies. The ability of certain remyelination promoting antibodies to target both membrane lipids and attached cytoskeletal proteins may significantly facilitate lesion clearance by the immune system and help to repopulate demyelinated areas with oligodendrocyte progenitor cells.

In summary, all remyelination promoting IgM mAbs bind to glycosphingolipids and potentially to glycoproteins at the cell surface of OPCs/OLs. It remains elusive whether effects seen *in vivo* and *in vitro* are mediated through binding to cell-surface glycosphingolipids, glycoproteins and/or internal cytoskeletal structures. Given the fact that antibody repair is mediated by a single peripheral injection, it is possible that IgM-induced repair mechanism may also be mediated by peripheral factors that seep into the CNS.

2.2.4   Low Amounts of rHIgM22 are Effective to Stimulate Remyelination in TMEV-Infected Animals

The effective dose of rHIgM22 to stimulate spinal cord remyelination in TMEV-infected mice is as low as 500 ng per mouse when administered i.p. in a single bolus injection. Remyelination was completed five weeks after the IgM injection. Higher antibody doses (up to 1000 fold) were not more effective in stimulating remyelination (19). It has been assumed that this is the limitation of the model during the chronic axonal phase of the disease. In addition, multiple antibody doses of rHIgM22 in TMEV-infected mice were not more effective compared to a single antibody dose.

In summary, rHIgM22 is a highly potent therapeutic in mice, mediates its effects within weeks and causes long-lasting tissue repair. It also suggests a molecular and cellular memory effect long after destruction of the antibody.

2.2.5   The Integrity of the IgM Molecule is Required to Stimulate Remyelination

Chemical or enzymatical cleavage of rHIgM22 into pseudo-IgGs resulted in lack of efficacy for the antibody to stimulate remyelination. Similarly, switching the antibody class from IgM to IgG for the mouse monoclonal IgM 94.03 and the human antibody rHIgM22 led to antibodies that had effects similar to PBS and entirely different compared to the intact pentameric IgM molecule with respect to stimulation of remyelination. This may either suggest that antigen clustering on a single living cell or clustering of multiple cells by the IgM molecule is essential for its cellular effects.

26

3

Natural Antibodies and
Their Potential Beneficial or Deleterious Effects
in The Peripheral Nervous System

Elevated levels of certain immunoglobulins, termed autoantibodies targeting glycosphingolipids and the myelin protein MAG, are sometimes found
in peripheral neuropathies (144). The constant association of anti-
glycosphingolipid antibodies with peripheral nervous system (PNS) dy-
simmune neuropathies supports a pathogenic link between anti-
glycosphingolipid antibodies and neuropathy (e.g., Miller Fisher syndrome (MFS); Guillain-Barre syndrome (GBS); neuropathy associated with
IgM monoclonal gammopathy (PN+IgM); chronic inflammatory demyelinating polyneuropathy (CIDP)). This includes immunoglobulins of the
isotypes IgG, IgA and IgM. Anti-MAG antibodies and > 20 different glycosphingolipids have been associated with chronic and acute peripheral neu-
ropathic syndromes of including GM1b, GD1a, GM1, GalNAc-GD1a (acute
motor axonal neuropathy), GQ1b, GD3, GD1b, GT1a (sensory variants of
GBS) (144) and sulfatide (GBS, CIDP) (145).

In contrast to their suggested involvement in peripheral neuropathies, gangliosides promote neurite outgrowth and regeneration both *in
vivo* and *in vitro* (146). Clinical trials using purified gangliosides in neuromuscular disorders did not show sufficient efficacy but also did not give
rise to an immune response followed by increased pathology (147). Intra-
muscular doses of purified bovine ganglioside mixtures were used therapeutically for years throughout Europe, and it is widely believed that these protein-free sphingolipids are not antigenic and do not elicit immune-

mediated side-effects. Experimentally, several studies failed to show that gangliosides enhance autoimmune demyelination in the PNS (148) and did not induce neurological signs of neuropathies or neuropathological changes (149). In addition, passive transfer of anti-GM1 antibodies failed to transfer the disease (150). All of this argues against the hypothesis that antibodies targeting glycosphingolipids are involved in the pathogenesis of peripheral neuropathies.

Interestingly, antibodies associated with peripheral neuropathies can bind to similar or identical antigens as remyelination-promoting antibodies and can be of IgM isotype similar to remyelination-promoting antibodies. At least some antibodies associated with peripheral neuropathies may act through complement fixation (151), which results in pore formation and cellular destruction after plasma-membrane binding. In contrast to these antibodies, the remyelination-promoting antibody rHIgM22 does not fix complement and does not target Schwann cells or peripheral nerves (unpublished data). Toxicology studies in primates and rodents using 1000-fold higher amounts of rHIgM22 than the therapeutic dose demonstrated no pathological effects in the PNS. Lack of antibody binding to peripheral nerves, however, suggests that rHIgM22 does not stimulate remyelination in the peripheral nervous system.

Unlike rHIgM22, remyelination-promoting antibodies O4 (sulfatide), O1 (galactosylceramide) and HNK1 (anti-SGPG, MAG) do bind to cell surface antigens on Schwann cells. It has not been determined whether these antibodies stimulate remyelination in the PNS. Surprisingly, antibodies associated with peripheral neuropathies target the same antigens as the mentioned promoters of remyelination (see above). The different outcome of various antibodies targeting identical antigens on myelinating oligodendrocytes versus Schwann cells raises the question whether antibodies associated with peripheral neuropathies actively exacerbate the disease course or merely represent a bystander effect. Generation of anti-sphingolipid antibodies may occur after the axonal and myelin destruction due to increasing amounts of cellular debris.

Given the number of different diseases covered under the umbrella of "peripheral neuropathies" and their individual complexity, it is extremely difficult to extrapolate which antibodies actively participate in the pathogenesis of different neuropathies based on clinical studies using immunosuppressive and immunomodulatory drugs. However, the efficacy of current immune therapies such as rituximab, prednisolone and cyclophosphamide in neuropathies with anti-MAG IgM antibodies remains unproven (152). Plasma exchange (PE) seems to be effective in patients with paraproteinemic neuropathies associated with high IgG or IgA antibodies but not IgM antibodies (153). Similarly, corticosteroids, when administered in monotheraphy, were not effective in IgM-associated neuropathies (154). In support of suggested differences between different antibody isotypes in paraproteinemic neuropathies, IgM-associated distal demyelinating symmetric neuropathies respond rather poorly to immunosuppressive therapy (155).

We conclude that IgMs targeting sphingolipids are unlikely pathogenic. However, it remains elusive whether remyelination promoting IgM antibodies O4, O1 and HNK-1 are beneficial for patients with peripheral neuropathies.

4

Immunotherapies using
Conventional Antibodies and Natural Antibodies
in Neurodegenerative Diseases

The level of progress in using immunotherapeutic approaches to combat neurodegenerative disorders depends on the specific disease and the cellular or extracellular location of the toxic protein aggregate. Alzheimer's disease (AD) has been the target of intensive work in several ongoing clinical trials with the goal to clear aggregated amyloid beta (Aβ) protein by immunotherapy in the extracellular space of CNS cells. Other neurodegenerative disorders including Parkinson's disease (PD) and other synucleinopathies, Huntington Disease and amyotrophic lateral sclerosis (ALS) were excluded as targetable diseases by immunotherapeutic approaches due to their (non-targetable) intracellular localization of toxic protein aggregates. This point of view changed through recent discoveries in studies showing cell surface exposure of aggregated toxic α-synuclein and tau isoforms. Most importantly, recent studies show exocytosis of aggregated proteins into the extracellular space with antigens accessible by antibodies.

4.1   Immunotherapy in AD

AD is becoming progressively prevalent as the global population ages with currently ~44 million victims of AD dementia worldwide (156). Pathological hallmarks of AD are extracellular deposits of Aβ in "amyloid plaques" in brain parenchyma and arterioles and intracellular hyperphosphorylated neurofibrillary tangles consisting of the cytoskeletal protein tau. AD is also characterized by extensive loss of neurons/synapses in temporal and cortical regions, mitochondrial oxidative damage, synaptic loss, proliferation and activation of astrocytes and microglia (157–159). Currently, there is no treatment available to cure or prevent AD.

Active and Passive Immunizations

Active and passive immunizations are under investigation for AD, each with its own advantages and disadvantages.

Active immunizations are based on the antigen combined with a strong immune-activating adjuvant to ensure high antibody titers. They engage the cellular and humoral immune system including B-cell and T-cell activation to stimulate antigen-specific antibody production. Active immunizations can induce long-lasting antibody productions while being very cost effective with small amounts of antigen administered and only few doctor visits. Unfortunately, active immunizations bear the risk of T-cell activation with possible subsequent deleterious pro-inflammatory cytokine production especially in cases where T-cells recognize the antigen as a self-protein. Furthermore, potential adverse or beneficial immune responses decay slowly over time, which can be problematic in cases with severe side effects. Active immunization results in a broad polyclonal antibody response with multiple different antibodies targeting multiple epitopes on single antigens. This approach typically guarantees antibody binding to multiple antigen isoforms (e.g. monomeric, oligomeric and fibrillar Aβ peptides) but is not suitable to eliminate specific isoforms within the circulation.

Passive immunotherapies are based on direct injections of monoclonal antibodies into the host without raising an immune response with subsequent antibody production. Advantages of passive immunotherapies are the possibility to target specific isoforms of the antigen (e.g. fibrillar Aβ but not monomeric Aβ) and to stop adverse reactions immediately. Disadvantages are use of expensive humanized antibodies with usually monthly injections for chronic diseases. Repeated dosing bears the risk of neutralizing antibody production in the host, which may eliminate or lower the effective antibody concentration required for a therapeutic effect.

Animal Models

Active immunizations with aggregated Aβ peptide in animal models of the disease before or after plaque deposition had an amazing beneficial effect on plaque pathology and an even more pronounced effect on the behavioral outcome (160, 161).

Similarly to active immunizations, **passive immunizations** using monoclonal antibodies targeting Aβ in animal models of AD reduced plaque pathology and improved the behavioral outcome in animals (162, 163). Even single antibody doses had measureable effects on behavior (164). Interestingly, the behavioral effects were not directly connected to Aβ plaque pathology. This suggested that (very small) soluble Aβ aggregates but not (large) plaque-like aggregates are responsible for the animals' behavioral deficits. However, levels of soluble Aβ measured by ELISA did not correlate with the strongly improved cognitive outcome in mice. Rare but highly toxic oligomeric Aβ aggregates difficult to detect by ELISA were postulated to explain the results (165). Phagocytosis of antibody-tagged Aβ aggregates through activated microglia and monocytes served as a possible explanation for the cognitive improvements in animals (166). However, Fab-fragments of antibodies lacking the Fc portion believed to be essential for antibody-stimulated phagocytosis resulted in identical plaque clearance in mice (167). This demonstrated that the antibodies Fc portion is not important for the behavioral improvement in mice and that antibody-stimulated phagocytosis by microglia/monocytes is unlikely involved in the process. Another hypothesis, commonly referred to as the "**peripheral sink hypothesis**", suggested that antibodies targeting the Aβ peptide in the blood draw soluble Aβ from the brain to the blood and thus reducing levels of aggregated Aβ in the CNS. This hypothesis is based on a potential equilibrium between soluble Aβ forms in the periphery and aggregated Aβ plaques in the brain, where Aβ can easily be tagged by antibodies and thus marked for destruction by the immune system.

Human Trials

Several different types of Aβ immunotherapies were investigated since the successful outcome in animal models including active and passive immunization strategies with either synthetic Aβ peptides, monoclonal antibodies targeting the Aβ peptide or IVIgG (168).

Active Aβ Immunotherapy

The first clinical trial AN1792 using active Aβ vaccine (Aβ1-42 combined with the strong adjuvant saporin and polysorbate 80) was halted in 2002 due to development of meningoencephalitis in 6 % of the moderate to severe AD patients (169). About 19 % of patients produced anti- Aβ antibodies that targeted plaques and vascular amyloid in human brain sections. Based on autopsy material from few responders of the Aβ vaccine in the years following the trial it was concluded that the Aβ deposition was reduced in specific brain regions without improving cognitive function (170). This result indicated that plaque removal at late disease-stages with already formed neurofibrillar tangles and substantial neuronal loss has no obvious beneficial effect. Surprisingly, dystrophic neurites and tau protein aggregates in neuropil threads were reduced by AN1792 but levels of toxic intracellular tau aggregates were unchanged (171, 172). It can be concluded that opsonization and removal of extracellular tau aggregates has little overall effect on Alzheimer disease pathogenesis at least during late disease stages. The results also suggest that there is no fast (not within years) equilibrium between intracellular tau aggregates, accessible cell surface tau isoforms and extracellular tau deposits, which indirectly contradicts the "peripheral sink hypothesis". While specific reasons for the development of meningoencephalitis are undetermined in the AN1792 trial, substantial efforts were undertaken to test passive immunotherapies using humanized anti- Aβ monoclonal antibodies to avoid autoimmune-like reactions. In addition, second generation active vaccines were developed that focus on the Aβ B-cell epitope (first 15 amino acids of the N-terminal part of the Aβ1-42 peptide) while avoiding the Aβ T-cell epitope (mid-region and C-terminal part of Aβ1-42) (173).

Two active Aβ vaccines containing short N-terminal Aβ peptides linked to inactivated diphtheria toxin (Aβ 1-7, trial ACC-001) respective bacteriophage QB virus particles (Aβ 1-7, trial CAD106) plus adjuvant are currently tested in clinical trials for patients with mild (CAD106) and mild to moderate AD (ACC-001). The AD vaccine *Vanutide cridificar* (trial ACC-001) was tested in multiple phase II trials. Official results have not been published in peer-reviewed journals. However, two serious adverse effects were reported by *Arai et al* (2013) at the AD Association International Conference 2013 in Boston (Abstract No. P1-338) with one patient developing contusion, cholecystitis infective, and duodenal ulcer and a second patient developed angina pectoris. In August 2013 *Pfizer* listed *Vanutide cridificar* (trial ACC-001) as discontinued from clinical development. (http://www.alzforum.org/therapeutics/vanutide-cridificar).

Phase II CAD106 trials were recently completed and the data analyses are pending. The CAD106 first in human study demonstrated a favorable safety profile and promising antibody responses (174). Other approaches using active vaccination are mimotopic/affitopic peptides that mimic (one) epitopes on the N-terminal part of the Aβ1-42 peptide. A phase 1 study tested subcutaneous vaccine administration (AD02) alone and with aluminium hydroxide adjuvant in patients with mild to moderate AD demonstrating a favorable safety and tolerability profile without cases of meningoencephalitis (175). The following phase II trial of AD02 in 332 patients with early AD as diagnosed by episodic memory deficit and hippocampal atrophy was conducted between 2010 and 2013. At a press briefing in June 2014, AFFiRiS showed limited trial data suggesting that AD02 had not reached either primary or secondary outcome measures. A follow-up study is still listed as enrolling (http://www.alzforum.org/therapeutics/affitope-ad02).

Passive Aβ Immunotherapy

Unfortunately, treatment with the monoclonal antibody Bapineuzumab resulted in meningoencephalitis, vasogenic edema and microhemorrhages (176). Bapineuzumab targets the extreme N-terminal 5 residues of the Aβ peptide and binds primarily to misfolded Aβ present in the brain. A phase III trial using Babineuzumab was halted because it did not affect cognitive function (177). Different from Babineuzumab, the monoclonal antibody Solanezumab selectively binds to soluble Aβ with little to no affinity towards fibrillar Aβ isoforms. Solanezumab was expected to show less CNS adverse events than Bapineuzumab. Indeed, Solanezumab showed good safety and some cognitive effects in mild but not moderate AD patients (178). However, two independent phase III trials using Solanezumab missed the goal of significantly slowing progression in AD. Similarly, the monoclonal antibody Ponezumab showed good safety data but did not affect levels of cognitive impairment compared to control groups and trials were discontinued (179). Ponezumab targets the C-terminal part of mis-folded Aβ peptide.

IVIgG Treatment in AD

Recent failures of passive Aβ immunotherapies in AD patients raised the question whether polyclonal antibody approaches like IVIgG may be more successful by simultaneously targeting monomeric, oligomeric and fibrillar Aβ and tau protein isoforms. Furthermore, IVIgG preparations likely contain antibodies directed against various nucleic acid-, lipid-, protein- and carbohydrate epitopes present on biomolecules that may be involved in AD pathogenesis.

A retrospective case-control analysis in non-Alzheimer disease patients 65 years or older treated with IVIgG versus untreated non-Alzheimer disease control patients of similar age demonstrated a 42 % lower risk in IVIgG treated patients of being diagnosed with AD (180). This result suggested a prophylactic effect of IVIgG in AD before patients become symptomatic. It was unclear whether IVIgG treatment has a beneficial effect post diagnosis in mild, moderate or severe AD patients. Pilot studies using IVIgG preparations for the treatment of mild to moderate AD patients suggested stabilization of cognitive functions (181, 182). The positive outcome of both studies was repeated in a phase II trial with the IVIgG Gammagard.[1] Unfortunately, a phase II AD trial using the IVIgG Octagam found no evidence for slowing down disease progression (183). Interestingly, no increase in serum Aβ1-40 was found in Octagam IVIgG treated patients, which was in contrast to reported pilot studies. Increased serum Aβ1-40 levels in pilot studies were interpreted as an IVIgG-stimulated efflux of brain Aβ isoforms into the peripheral circulation. A phase III AD trial using the IVIgG Gammagard confirmed the negative outcome from the phase II Octagam trial and reported no evidence for slowing down disease progression (Medpage Today: AD: IVIg Fails in Trial. http://bit.ly/IVIgG_Trial) (184). Two AD-related IVIgG trials are still in progress. Flebogamma (Grifols Biologicals) is currently in a phase III AD trial and NewGam (Octapharma) is being investigated by Sutter

---

[1] Science Daily: Results Of 9-Month Phase II Study Of Gammagard Intravenous Immuno-globulin. http://bit.ly/IVIgG_Gammagard; Medpage Today: IVIg Stops AD in Its Tracks. http://bit.ly/IVIgG_Alzheimer

Health in a phase II trial to determine its effects in AD patients with amnestic mild cognitive impairment (MCI).

Reasons for the different outcome of IVIgG in AD studies are unclear. The higher statistical power of the larger phase II Octagam and phase III Gammagard AD trials compared to small pilot studies indicated no beneficial effect of IVIgG at least during later stages of AD. IVIgG may, however, have a prophylactic effect before onset of symptoms in patients at risk of being diagnosed with AD. A general problem in the comparison of studies using different IVIG preparations are potential differences in the IVIgG composition that may lead to unknown effects on the study outcome. It has been assumed that Aβ and tau protein reactivity by IVIgG antibodies is an essential prerequisite for a potential beneficial outcome in AD trials. The IVIgG preparation used in the Octagam trial was shown to contain at least some antibodies targeting Aβ (185). However, different antibody concentrations for Aβ (186, 187) and tau (188) were detected in different IVIgG batches used in AD studies.

Critical remark: Use of IVIgG for the treatment of AD and other neurodegenerative disorders appears to correlate (besides limited serum resources and other factors) with lack of profound knowledge with respect to disease pathogenesis and targetable pathogenic factors. IVIgG preparations likely include antibodies for identified or non-identified disease-causing agents, however, at low or very low concentrations while the vast majority of immunoglobulins are off-target. It remains elusive whether effective concentrations of disease relevant antibodies in IVIgG preparations are high enough to show reproducible therapeutic effects, particularly with lack of consistency in IVIgG preparations. Different from immune-mediated and/or peripheral disorders only small amounts of therapeutic antibodies present in IVIgG preparations are able to cross the blood brain barrier to target their CNS antigen. The discrepancy in required therapeutic concentrations of antibodies targeting Aβ, tau and other CNS disease causing agents becomes even more apparent if we assume a neutralizing role of antibodies in stoichiometric or close to stoichiometric ratios relative to Aβ or tau concentrations.

NAbs for the Treatment of AD

Polyclonal NAbs targeting Aβ peptides (Aβ-NAbs) exist at low concentration in serum and cerebrospinal fluid (CSF) of healthy individuals and are reduced in AD patients (181, 189, 190). Aβ-NAbs are therefore present in IVIgG preparations. Aβ-NAbs from sera of healthy donors and IVIgG preparations are considered natural antibodies because none of the donors were immunized with (aggregated) Aβ isoforms. Previous studies on NAbs postulated that Aβ-NAbs may serve as surveillance molecules to eliminate toxic aggregates before they can elicit a deleterious response. Human Aβ-NAbs were detected by ELISA and were of IgM- or IgG-isotype. The specific activity of IgM Aβ-NAbs was 2.5-fold higher than the IgG Aβ-NAbs. This interesting result was confirmed in a commercial IVIgG preparation (Pentaglobin, Biotest, Germany) containing both IgM and IgG antibodies. The specific activities of IgM and IgG Aβ-NAbs were 63 and 17 titer units/mg (191). In mouse models of AD, murine IgM Aβ-NAbs demonstrated cerebral Aβ clearance without crossing the blood brain barrier (192).

Epitope specificity of Aβ-NAbs towards small linear Aβ peptides present in sera of healthy donors and IVIgG preparations demonstrated a 20 % increased N-terminal preference (amino acids 1-7) relative to the Aβ central regions (amino acids 15–25) (191). This outcome was in contrast to the Aβ reactivity of Aβ-NAbs from healthy patient sera towards oligomeric but not fibrillar Aβ1-42 aggregates (193, 194). In epitope-mapping studies Aβ-NAbs mainly targeted central or C-terminal regions of Aβ1-42 starting with amino acid 28 (193, 194). The conformational specificity of Aβ-NAbs is in contrast to most monoclonal antibodies including Bapineuzumab and Solanezumab which target linear epitopes in N-terminal (Bapineuzumab) or central regions (Solanezumab) of Aβ (for review see (195).

Similarly, active immunizations like AN1792 generated primarily antibodies targeting the accessible N-terminal part of aggregated Aβ1-42 (196). Differences in epitope specificity of potential therapeutic antibodies may be crucial for their outcome in human trials because soluble, oligomeric Aβ isoforms are expected to be neurotoxic whereas insoluble, fibrillar Aβ aggregates or monomeric Aβ peptides are expected to be inert. The epitope specificity of Aβ-NAbs towards oligomeric Aβ isoforms may also indicate that Aβ-NAbs are unable to clear CNS resident Aβ plaques consisting of mainly fibrillar Aβ. This concept can, however, be questioned by the existence of a kinetically reasonable equilibrium between monomeric, oligomeric and fibrillar Aβ isoforms, which is the fundamental basis of the "peripheral sink hypothesis". Without this postulated equilibrium between different Aβ isoforms in the CNS and the peripheral circulation antibody-mediated reduction of soluble Aβ monomers/oligomers in the periphery will have no effect on oligomeric or fibrillar Aβ deposits in the brain. It would also mean that epitope specificity of potentially therapeutic antibodies towards certain structural motifs/Aβ isoforms is insignificant because all isoforms are principally convertible into each other when "pulled out" of the equilibrium through antibody binding.

IgM NAbs with the ability to target and enzymatically cleave β-amyloid have been isolated from a patient with Waldenström Macroglobulinemia (197) and are promising candidates in battling AD. A more recent publication from the same group reported a more specific metal-dependent amyloid β-degrading catalytic antibody construct (198).

In summary, NAbs may represent a promising class of molecules to combat AD when used in sufficient concentrations. Similar to conventional antibodies, NAbs may impact the disease course when used in sufficient concentrations at earlier disease stages. It is still controversial whether the antibody's isotype impacts its efficacy to clear CNS Aβ aggregates and improve cognitive scores in AD. However, recent studies highlight IgM NAbs as potential alternatives to IgG NAbs in combating AD.

Reasons for Failure of Therapeutics Including Immunotherapies in AD

Drug development for AD has been proven to be very difficult. Five drugs have been FDA approved for AD including four cholinesterase inhibitors (tacrine, donepezil, rivastigmine, galantamine) and one N-methyl-D-aspartate (NMDA) receptor antagonist (memantine). Tacrine was withdrawn from the US market in May 2012 due to safety concerns with several instances of clinically apparent, acute liver injury (199). No new treatments have been approved since 2003. From 2002 until 2012 both small molecules and immunotherapies (244 unique compounds of disease modifying or symptomatic agents) failed in 413 trials (124 Phase I, 206 Phase II, 83 Phase III) to show efficacy over placebo, due to unacceptable toxicity or challenges in trial execution. Trial conduct failure may be due to lack of decline in the placebo group, no effects in active-comparator arms of the study, or excessive measurement variability (200-203). 145 out of 221 human trials in AD (between 2002 and 2012) applying disease-modifying agents used some Aβ isoform (monomeric, oligomeric or fibrillar isoform) as pharmacological target (202). It should be emphasized that no class of agent has shown efficacy for targeting Aβ isoforms in human trials while animal models of amyloidosis demonstrated substantial pathological and behavioral benefits from anti-Aβ drugs (202). This data not only highlights a "translational gap" between the human situation and existing mouse amyloidosis models, which is likely a major reason for lack of progress in drug development for AD but furthermore questions the "unique" role of Aβ in disease progression and for drug development. Too small amounts of hydrophilic compounds crossing the BBB are another likely reason for lack of efficacy in human trials (see BBB section below). While this is true for large protein based agents (antibodies = immunotherapies) at least some small molecules used in human trials were lipophilic enough to ensure sufficient CNS concentrations. Surprisingly, all agents tested in human trials in between 2002 and 2012 were not FDA approved (with the exception of memantine) irrespective of the physico-chemical properties of the agents used.

While potential therapeutics are applicable to all ages of transgenic mice human treatments were started too late in the progression of AD. Treatment at late stages of the disease may not overcome the deficits of neuronal loss similar to chronic stages in other neurological diseases. The major difficulty is, however, to identify patients early enough in the disease course. In addition, early stage AD patients may lack disease symptoms and compliance in taking medications with potentially severe side effects might be low.

Animal models more predictive of success for human trials that fully represent human disease pathology are clearly necessary. Current animal models typically present one or two aspects of AD pathology (204–206). Transgenic mice expressing tau protein or tau/APP mutations are expected to be suitable models for testing cytoskeletal and tau-oriented therapeutics (207, 208), while transgenic animals harboring presenilin mutations may be more appropriate models for testing γ-secretase inhibitors (209). In addition, diversification of therapeutic targets in AD and combined therapeutic approaches with multiple disease pathways affected/blocked may improve the success rate in human trials.

4.2   Immunotherapies for α-synucleinopathies Including Idiopathic Parkinson's Disease, Dementia with Lewy Bodies and Parkinson's Disease Dementia

Lewy body diseases are among the most common neurodegenerative diseases followed by AD and vascular dementia. Synucleinopathies also known as Lewy body diseases (LBDs), are characterized by degeneration of the dopaminergic system, motor alterations, cognitive impairment, and formation of Lewy bodies (LBs) and/or Lewy neurites (210, 211). Synucleinopathies include Parkinson's disease (PD) (including idiopathic PD), Diffuse Lewy Body Disease (DLBD) also known as Dementia with Lewy Bodies (DLB), Lewy body variant of AD (LBV), Combined AD and PD, pure autonomic failure and multiple system atrophy (MSA e.g., Olivopontocerebellar Atrophy, Striatonigral Degeneration and Shy-Drager Syndrome). Several nonmotor signs and symptoms are thought to be harbingers for synucleinopathies in the prodromal phase of the diseases (i.e, the presymptomatic, subclinical, preclinical, or premotor period). Such early signs include, for example, REM sleep behavior disorder (RBD), loss of smell and constipation (212). Lewy body diseases continue to be a common cause for movement disorders and cognitive deterioration in the aging population (213).

The major pathological feature of PD is the death of dopaminergic neurons in the substantia nigra, while dementia with Lewy bodies (DLB) and PD dementia additionally include death of cholinergic neurons in the basal forebrain (214, 215).

Several studies implicated a central role for α-synuclein in PD pathogenesis. α-synuclein can aggregate into insoluble fibrils and accumulates in LBs (216, 217). Mutations in the α-synuclein gene co-segregate with rare familial forms of Parkinsonism (218, 219). Overexpression of α-synuclein in transgenic mice mimics several pathological aspects of Lewy body disease (220). In addition, it has been suggested that soluble oligomers of α-synuclein may be neurotoxic (221, 222).

Animal models

The fact that α-synuclein aggregates can be exocytosed, localize at the plasma membrane and propagate extracellularly, provided a rationale for immunotherapeutic approaches (223). Neurons and glia are able to propagate the disease through endocytosis of the toxic α-synuclein-containing particles and subsequent formation of intracellular inclusion bodies (223). Interestingly, recent animal studies demonstrated clearing of intraneuronal α-synuclein aggregates combined with memory improvements by immunotherapy using the α-synuclein targeting antibodies 9E4 and 1H7 (224). Antibody 9E4 targets amino acids 118-126 on α-synuclein and 1H7 targets amino acids 91-99 on α-synuclein. The study also suggested that the antibodies isotype may be important for the behavioral outcome. While antibodies 9E4 and 1H7 (both IgG1 isotype) improved mater maze performance in mice demonstrated antibody 5D12 lack of efficacy in behavioral tests. 5D12 targets the identical α-synuclein motif as 9E4 but belongs to the IgG2 antibody isotype. Interestingly, the animal study also included a modified antibody termed 5C1 (isotype IgG1) targeting identical amino acids as 9E4. While 5C1 failed in behavioral tests it reduced ELADW-105 positive neuritic dystrophy to levels similar to antibodies 9E4, 1H7 but not 5D12 (patent US20130108546 A1: Humanized Antibodies That Recognize α-Synuclein). This data suggested a disconnection between neuropathological outcomes and improved cognitive scores. In trangenic mice, antibody 9E4 also reduced the area of neuropil by 43% in neocortex and by 40% in basal ganglia as compared to control. The 9E4 antibody preserved synaptophysin and MAP2 in neocortex and basal ganglia (patent US20130108546 A1: Humanized Antibodies That Recognize α-Synuclein). Antibody 9E4 has also been reported to reduce levels of a C-terminally truncated form of α-synculein that is considered neurotoxic, as well as α-synculein propagation from cell to cell, and to improve behavioral endpoints (224-226).

Human Trials

Prothena and Roche initiated a Phase I clinical trial for PRX002 for the treatment of PD in April 2014. PRX002 is a humanized IgG1 monoclonal antibody of the murine antibody 9E4 directed against aggregated α-synuclein. Results of the Phase I trial demonstrated that PRX002 was safe and well tolerated. Further, results from this study showed that administration of PRX002 leads to mean reduction of free serum α-synuclein levels of up to 96% ($p < 0.00001$). Reduction of free serum α-synuclein was shown to be robust, rapid and dose-dependent after just a single dose.

NAbs as Potential Biomarkers in PD

The presence of natural antibodies targeting α-synuclein has been demonstrated in patient sera from familial and sporadic PD as well as healthy control sera (227). Multiepitopic autoantibodies against α-synuclein are detectable in 65% of all patients (228). α-synuclein NAb levels were low in sera from PD patients compared to healthy controls and suggested a potential use of NAbs as diagnostic biomarkers (229). However, a recent study reported strong inconsistencies in the detection of ELISA-based α-Syn-nAbs levels in serum and cerebrospinal fluid of 66 PD patients and 69 healthy controls (230). While α-synuclein-NAbs levels may represent a potential PD biomarker, several methodological issues have to be considered to increase reproducibility of α-synuclein-NAbs findings. Importantly, depending on posttranslational modifications, aggregation status and environmental factors α-synuclein oligomers/fibrils will have different conformations and therefore changed accessibility for targeting antibodies with hidden and newly formed epitopes (neoepitopes) (231). So far, serum α-synuclein-NAbs do not interact with oligomeric, fibrillar or heterogeneous oligomeric α-synuclein (232). Epitope specificity for α-synuclein-NAbs still has to be determined.

   It remains unclear whether α-synuclein-NAbs can either be used as viable biomarkers or as potential blocking agents to inhibit cell-to-cell propagation of toxic α-synuclein oligomers.

4.3   Immunotherapies for Creuzfeld-Jakob Disease and Prions

Prion diseases are untreatable and fatal neurodegenerative disorders caused by the conversion and deposition of the native prion protein termed PrPC in its aggregated pathological isoform PrPSc. The native prion protein PrPC is ubiquitously expressed on the cell surface of neuronal cells and leukocytes. Pathological hallmarks of the disease are CNS restricted depositions of aggregated and infectious PrPSc, neuronal death and vacuolization of grey matter. These effects are typically combined with inflammatory processes leading to astrogliosis and microglial activation.

Animal Models

Immunotherapeutic approaches using monoclonal antibodies *in vivo* and *in vitro* suppressed prion infectivity, peripheral prion replication and delayed the disease onset (233, 234). Antibodies ICSM35 and ICSM18 targeting PrP91-110 (ICSM35) respective PrP146-159 (ICSM18) of murine PrP^C inhibited splenic PrP^{Sc} propagation and substantially extended life-span when administered intraperitoneally. It is of note that passive immunization of anti-PrP antibodies had no effect on survival after clinical signs had developed (234). Transgenic expression of the μ heavy chain of the prion specific monoclonal antibody 6H4, which targets PrP144-152 in PrP$^{+/-}$ mice, completely abolished prion infection after intraperitoneal PrP^{Sc} administration (235).

In cell culture models prion infectivity was most successfully inhibited by prion specific Fab fragments targeting PrP132-156, followed by Fab fragments targeting PrP95-103. Antibodies targeting the very C-terminal region of the prion protein PrP220-231 had significantly smaller effects on inhibition of PrP^{Sc} propagation compared to antibodies targeting the Helix1 containing region (PrP143-153) of the murine prion protein (233). Low affinity antibodies against PrP29–37 and PrP72–86 were ineffective to influence PrP^{Sc} propagation *in vitro* (236).

Given the fact that the physiological function of the cellular prion protein is still undetermined, immunizations with PrP^C-specific antibodies may lead to PrP^C depletion with unknown consequences. In fact, a recent study showed that PrP^C-specific antibodies could trigger apoptosis of neural cells through PrP^C crosslinking (237). So far, all immunotherapeutic approaches using monoclonal antibodies for the treatment of prion diseases are yet to show efficacy in patients (238).

NAbs as Potential Blocking Agents in Prion Diseases

Natural IgG autoantibodies present in the CSF and serum from healthy individuals were identified that block prion fibril formation and neurotoxicity *in vitro* (239). IgG PrP-NAbs were isolated from IVIgG preparations and targeted PrP106-126 within the prion protein. Similar to conventional antibodies identified to block prion propagation IgG PrP-NAbs targeted the Proteinase K-resistant central core of the prion protein ~ PrP90-144 that likely converts to β-sheet rich structures upon prion protein aggregation

(240). Thus, no obvious differences between IgG PrP-NAbs and conventional antibodies were detected with respect to structural prion elements or antibody isotypes used to target the prion protein.

Results from PrP-NAbs underline the potential of natural autoantibodies for the treatment of prion diseases. However, more studies are necessary to confirm a positive effect of NAbs in cell culture models and animals on prion propagation. In analogy to other neurodegenerative diseases, the potential clinical application may be most successful when applied at early stages of the disease. In addition, the amount of blocking antibodies (NAbs and conventional antibodies) required for potential therapeutic effects in prion diseases is expected to be close to stoichiometric ratios relative to the amount of toxic prion aggregates present.

5

The Blood Brain Barrier and Its Impact on Treatment Strategies for Neurological Diseases

The blood brain barrier (BBB) controls the transport of hydrophilic substances (e.g. antibodies) from the periphery into the CNS. It is therefore the major obstacle for brain and spinal cord delivery of antibodies when injected peripherally. The extent of BBB leakage is expected to be different in neuroinflammatory compared to neurodegenerative diseases with higher rates of BBB permeability under inflammatory conditions. In general, dysfunction of the BBB is a major hallmark of MS (241, 242) and has been demonstrated in different presentations of the disease including chronic-progressive MS (243) and acute MS plaques (244). In contrast, most studies measuring serum albumin levels in the CSF of AD patients show normal albumin levels similar to those in healthy patients (245).

Animal studies using monoclonal antibodies for the treatment of neurologic diseases reported 0.01 to 0.4 % of injected antibodies to cross the BBB with very little impact of the animal model (246–249) or the antibody isotype used (Warrington *et al*, unpublished data). The low amount of antibodies crossing the BBB may at least in part be responsible for the low clinical success rate of Aβ targeting antibodies in AD patients.

A recent option to increase BBB crossover of antibodies is to target receptors on the BBB for either transcytosis or active transport from the blood to the CNS. This approach increased the antibody penetration rate to 2-3 % relative to the injected dose (250) and may be sufficient to switch a clinically ineffective antibody to an effective one. More specifically, bispecific IgG molecules were developed that target the transferrin receptor with one Fab and the β-secretase involved in CNS Aβ production with the other Fab. This approach resulted in significantly reduced Aβ levels in the brain (251). Another approach that increased the antibodies BBB crossover was to fuse the antibody with the receptor-binding domain of apolipoprotein B and E (252). Future studies are required to potentially translate these findings into the clinic for the benefit of patients with CNS diseases.

6

Conclusions

There is a need to identify new treatment strategies for basically all neuro-logic diseases including MS and neurodegenerative diseases. In demye-linating diseases like MS the therapeutic focus should be on strategies that actively induce brain lesion repair and stimulation of remyelination. Tar-geting the immune system did not prevent or reverse long term disabili-ties. Future prospects for remyelination therapies are encouraging. Poten-tial combinatorial therapeutic approaches could include agents that target the immune system to eliminate deleterious immune system-mediated in-jury and perhaps NAbs that stimulate remyelination. Indeed, human monoclonal IgMs that target the CNS may enhance the permissive envi-ronment for regenerating lost myelin. The very low amount of the human antibody rHIgM22 necessary for stimulation of remyelination in mice and an open BBB during acute phases of the human disease are encouraging and give hope for MS patients.

Different from MS, the perspective of antibody therapy in neuro-degenerative diseases is less promising. Major obstacles are the BBB and cell intrinsic death programs activated (synucleinopathies, prion diseases) before antibodies can tag and destroy toxic protein aggregates. Therapeu-tic antibody-mediated effects in genetic forms of neurodegenerative dis-eases mentioned above are rather unlikely, because all neuronal cells bear the deleterious mutation causing cell intrinsic toxic protein aggregates. Cell to cell propagation of toxic protein aggregates is not required to cause substantial cell death in familial cases because all cells are able to produce misfolded, toxic proteins without external stimuli. Therapeutic antibodies may slow down disease progression by preventing spreading of toxic aggregates from cell to cell. The low amount of antibodies crossing the BBB combined with the fact that antibodies in neurodegenerative diseases most likely act like neutralizing agents in or close to stoichiometric ratios relative to the amount of protein aggregates, makes a therapeutic antibody approach inside the brain rather unlikely.

References

1. Merbl Y, Zucker-Toledano M, Quintana FJ, & Cohen IR (2007) Newborn humans manifest autoantibodies to defined self molecules detected by antigen microarray informatics. (Translated from eng) *J Clin Invest* 117(3):712-718 (in eng).

2. Avrameas S (1991) Natural autoantibodies: from 'horror autotoxicus' to 'gnothi seauton'. (Translated from eng) *Immunol Today* 12(5):154-159 (in eng).

3. Coutinho A, Kazatchkine MD, & Avrameas S (1995) Natural autoantibodies. (Translated from eng) *Curr Opin Immunol* 7(6):812-818 (in eng).

4. Dighiero G, *et al.* (1983) Murine hybridomas secreting natural monoclonal antibodies reacting with self antigens. (Translated from eng) *J Immunol* 131(5):2267-2272 (in eng).

5. Haspel MV, *et al.* (1983) Virus-induced autoimmunity: monoclonal antibodies that react with endocrine tissues. (Translated from eng) *Science* 220(4594):304-306 (in eng).

6. Haspel MV, *et al.* (1983) Multiple organ-reactive monoclonal autoantibodies. (Translated from eng) *Nature* 304(5921):73-76 (in eng).

7. Prabhakar BS, Saegusa J, Onodera T, & Notkins AL (1984) Lymphocytes capable of making monoclonal autoantibodies that react with multiple organs are a common feature of the normal B cell repertoire. (Translated from eng) *J Immunol* 133(6):2815-2817 (in eng).

8.   Satoh J, Prabhakar BS, Haspel MV, Ginsberg-Fellner F, & Notkins AL (1983) Human monoclonal autoantibodies that react with multiple endocrine organs. (Translated from eng) *N Engl J Med* 309(4):217-220 (in eng).

9.   Lacroix-Desmazes S, *et al.* (1998) Self-reactive antibodies (natural autoantibodies) in healthy individuals. (Translated from eng) *J Immunol Methods* 216(1-2):117-137 (in eng).

10.   Merbl Y, Zucker-Toledano M, Quintana FJ, & Cohen IR (2007) Newborn humans manifest autoantibodies to defined self molecules detected by antigen microarray informatics. (Translated from eng) *J Clin Invest* 117(3):712-718 (in eng).

11.   Avrameas S & Selmi C (2013) Natural autoantibodies in the physiology and pathophysiology of the immune system. (Translated from eng) *Journal of autoimmunity* 41:46-49 (in eng).

12.   Avrameas S & Ternynck T (1993) The natural autoantibodies system: between hypotheses and facts. (Translated from eng) *Mol Immunol* 30(12):1133-1142 (in eng).

13.   Brandlein S, *et al.* (2007) The human IgM antibody SAM-6 induces tumor-specific apoptosis with oxidized low-density lipoprotein. (Translated from eng) *Mol Cancer Ther* 6(1):326-333 (in eng).

14.   Pohle T, Brandlein S, Ruoff N, Muller-Hermelink HK, & Vollmers HP (2004) Lipoptosis: tumor-specific cell death by antibody-induced intracellular lipid accumulation. (Translated from eng) *Cancer Res* 64(11):3900-3906 (in eng).

15.   Rauschert N, *et al.* (2008) A new tumor-specific variant of GRP78 as target for antibody-based therapy. (Translated from eng) *Lab Invest* 88(4):375-386 (in eng).

16.   Vollmers HP & Brandlein S (2009) Natural antibodies and cancer. (Translated from eng) *N Biotechnol* 25(5):294-298 (in eng).

17.   Bieber AJ, *et al.* (2002) Human antibodies accelerate the rate of remyelination following lysolecithin-induced demyelination in mice. (Translated from eng) *Glia* 37(3):241-249 (in eng).

18.   Warrington AE, *et al.* (2000) Human monoclonal antibodies reactive to oligodendrocytes promote remyelination in a model of multiple sclerosis. (Translated from eng) *Proc Natl Acad Sci U S A* 97(12):6820-6825 (in eng).

19.   Warrington AE, *et al.* (2007) A recombinant human IgM promotes myelin repair after a single, very low dose. (Translated from eng) *J Neurosci Res* 85(5):967-976 (in eng).

20.   Hooijkaas H, van der Linde-Preesman AA, Benne S, & Benner R (1985) Frequency analysis of the antibody specificity repertoire of mitogen-reactive B cells and "spontaneously" occurring "background" plaque-forming cells in nude mice. (Translated from eng) *Cell Immunol* 92(1):154-162 (in eng).

21.   Van Oudenaren A, Haaijman JJ, & Benner R (1984) Frequencies of background cytoplasmic Ig-containing cells in various lymphoid organs of athymic and euthymic mice as a function of age and immune status. (Translated from eng) *Immunology* 51(4):735-742 (in eng).

22.   Baumgarth N, Herman OC, Jager GC, Brown L, & Herzenberg LA (1999) Innate and acquired humoral immunities to influenza virus are mediated by distinct arms of the immune system. (Translated from eng) *Proc Natl Acad Sci U S A* 96(5):2250-2255 (in eng).

23.   Choi YS & Baumgarth N (2008) Dual role for B-1a cells in immunity to influenza virus infection. (Translated from eng) *J Exp Med* 205(13):3053-3064 (in eng).

24.   Kroese FG, *et al.* (1989) Many of the IgA producing plasma cells in murine gut are derived from self-replenishing precursors in the peritoneal cavity. (Translated from eng) *Int Immunol* 1(1):75-84 (in eng).

25.   Stall AM, Wells SM, & Lam KP (1996) B-1 cells: unique origins and functions. (Translated from eng) *Semin Immunol* 8(1):45-59 (in eng).

26.   Roy B, *et al.* (2009) Somatic hypermutation in peritoneal B1b cells. (Translated from eng) *Mol Immunol* 46(8-9):1613-1619 (in eng).

27. Tumas-Brundage KM, *et al.* (2001) Predominance of a novel splenic B cell population in mice expressing a transgene that encodes multireactive antibodies: support for additional heterogeneity of the B cell compartment. (Translated from eng) *Int Immunol* 13(4):475-484 (in eng).

28. Baumgarth N (2011) The double life of a B-1 cell: self-reactivity selects for protective effector functions. (Translated from eng) *Nature reviews. Immunology* 11(1):34-46 (in eng).

29. Holodick NE, Tumang JR, & Rothstein TL (2010) Immunoglobulin secretion by B1 cells: differential intensity and IRF4-dependence of spontaneous IgM secretion by peritoneal and splenic B1 cells. (Translated from eng) *Eur J Immunol* 40(11):3007-3016 (in eng).

30. Masmoudi H, Mota-Santos T, Huetz F, Coutinho A, & Cazenave PA (1990) All T15 Id-positive antibodies (but not the majority of VHT15+ antibodies) are produced by peritoneal CD5+ B lymphocytes. (Translated from eng) *Int Immunol* 2(6):515-520 (in eng).

31. Tumang JR, Frances R, Yeo SG, & Rothstein TL (2005) Spontaneously Ig-secreting B-1 cells violate the accepted paradigm for expression of differentiation-associated transcription factors. (Translated from eng) *J Immunol* 174(6):3173-3177 (in eng).

32. Ha SA, *et al.* (2006) Regulation of B1 cell migration by signals through Toll-like receptors. (Translated from eng) *J Exp Med* 203(11):2541-2550 (in eng).

33. Kawahara T, Ohdan H, Zhao G, Yang YG, & Sykes M (2003) Peritoneal cavity B cells are precursors of splenic IgM natural antibody-producing cells. (Translated from eng) *J Immunol* 171(10):5406-5414 (in eng).

34. Murakami M, *et al.* (1994) Oral administration of lipopolysaccharides activates B-1 cells in the peritoneal cavity and lamina propria of the gut and induces autoimmune symptoms in an autoantibody transgenic mouse. (Translated from eng) *J Exp Med* 180(1):111-121 (in eng).

35. Nisitani S, Tsubata T, Murakami M, & Honjo T (1995) Administration of interleukin-5 or -10 activates peritoneal B-1 cells and

induces autoimmune hemolytic anemia in anti-erythrocyte autoantibody-transgenic mice. (Translated from eng) *Eur J Immunol* 25(11):3047-3052 (in eng).

36.   Griffin DO, Holodick NE, & Rothstein TL (2011) Human B1 cells are CD3-: A reply to "A human equivalent of mouse B-1 cells?" and "The nature of circulating CD27+CD43+ B cells". (Translated from eng) *J Exp Med* 208(13):2566-2569 (in eng).

37.   Landsteiner K (1947) The Specificity of Serological Reactions. *Harvard: Harvard University Press.*

38.   Kijanka G, *et al.* (2009) Rapid characterization of binding specificity and cross-reactivity of antibodies using recombinant human protein arrays. (Translated from eng) *J Immunol Methods* 340(2):132-137 (in eng).

39.   Dighiero G, Guilbert B, & Avrameas S (1982) Naturally occurring antibodies against nine common antigens in humans sera. II. High incidence of monoclonal Ig exhibiting antibody activity against actin and tubulin and sharing antibody specificities with natural antibodies. (Translated from eng) *J Immunol* 128(6):2788-2792 (in eng).

40.   Quan CP, Berneman A, Pires R, Avrameas S, & Bouvet JP (1997) Natural polyreactive secretory immunoglobulin A autoantibodies as a possible barrier to infection in humans. (Translated from eng) *Infect Immun* 65(10):3997-4004 (in eng).

41.   Marchalonis JJ, Adelman MK, Robey IF, Schluter SF, & Edmundson AB (2001) Exquisite specificity and peptide epitope recognition promiscuity, properties shared by antibodies from sharks to humans. (Translated from eng) *J Mol Recognit* 14(2):110-121 (in eng).

42.   Notkins AL (2004) Polyreactivity of antibody molecules. (Translated from eng) *Trends Immunol* 25(4):174-179 (in eng).

43.   Ichiyoshi Y & Casali P (1994) Analysis of the structural correlates for antibody polyreactivity by multiple reassortments of chimeric human immunoglobulin heavy and light chain V segments. (Translated from eng) *J Exp Med* 180(3):885-895 (in eng).

44. Martin T, Crouzier R, Weber JC, Kipps TJ, & Pasquali JL (1994) Structure-function studies on a polyreactive (natural) autoantibody. Polyreactivity is dependent on somatically generated sequences in the third complementarity-determining region of the antibody heavy chain. (Translated from eng) *J Immunol* 152(12):5988-5996 (in eng).

45. Polymenis M & Stollar BD (1994) Critical binding site amino acids of anti-Z-DNA single chain Fv molecules. Role of heavy and light chain CDR3 and relationship to autoantibody activity. (Translated from eng) *J Immunol* 152(11):5318-5329 (in eng).

46. Fernandez C, Alarcon-Riquelme ME, & Sverremark E (1997) Polyreactive binding of antibodies generated by polyclonal B cell activation. II. Crossreactive and monospecific antibodies can be generated from an identical Ig rearrangement by differential glycosylation. (Translated from eng) *Scand J Immunol* 45(3):240-247 (in eng).

47. Leibiger H, Wustner D, Stigler RD, & Marx U (1999) Variable domain-linked oligosaccharides of a human monoclonal IgG: structure and influence on antigen binding. (Translated from eng) *Biochem J* 338 (Pt 2):529-538 (in eng).

48. Leung SO, *et al.* (1995) Effect of VK framework-1 glycosylation on the binding affinity of lymphoma-specific murine and chimeric LL2 antibodies and its potential use as a novel conjugation site. (Translated from eng) *Int J Cancer* 60(4):534-538 (in eng).

49. Bosshard HR (2001) Molecular recognition by induced fit: how fit is the concept? (Translated from eng) *News Physiol Sci* 16:171-173 (in eng).

50. Wedemayer GJ, Patten PA, Wang LH, Schultz PG, & Stevens RC (1997) Structural insights into the evolution of an antibody combining site. (Translated from eng) *Science* 276(5319):1665-1669 (in eng).

51. James LC, Roversi P, & Tawfik DS (2003) Antibody multispecificity mediated by conformational diversity. (Translated from eng) *Science* 299(5611):1362-1367 (in eng).

52.   Margulies DH (2003) Molecular interactions: stiff or floppy (or somewhere in between?). (Translated from eng) *Immunity* 19(6):772-774 (in eng).

53.   Pashov A, *et al.* (2005) Antigenic properties of peptide mimotopes of HIV-1-associated carbohydrate antigens. (Translated from eng) *J Biol Chem* 280(32):28959-28965 (in eng).

54.   Luo P, Canziani G, Cunto-Amesty G, & Kieber-Emmons T (2000) A molecular basis for functional peptide mimicry of a carbohydrate antigen. (Translated from eng) *J Biol Chem* 275(21):16146-16154 (in eng).

55.   McMahon MJ & O'Kennedy R (2000) Polyreactivity as an acquired artefact, rather than a physiologic property, of antibodies: evidence that monoreactive antibodies may gain the ability to bind to multiple antigens after exposure to low pH. (Translated from eng) *J Immunol Methods* 241(1-2):1-10 (in eng).

56.   Zhang M & Carroll MC (2007) Natural antibody mediated innate autoimmune response. (Translated from eng) *Mol Immunol* 44(1-3):103-110 (in eng).

57.   Darley-Usmar V & Halliwell B (1996) Blood radicals: reactive nitrogen species, reactive oxygen species, transition metal ions, and the vascular system. (Translated from eng) *Pharm Res* 13(5):649-662 (in eng).

58.   Dimitrov JD, *et al.* (2006) Ferrous ions and reactive oxygen species increase antigen-binding and anti-inflammatory activities of immunoglobulin G. (Translated from eng) *J Biol Chem* 281(1):439-446 (in eng).

59.   Mihaylova NM, Dimitrov JD, Djoumerska-Alexieva IK, & Vassilev TL (2008) Inflammation-induced enhancement of IgG immuno-reactivity. (Translated from eng) *Inflamm Res* 57(1):1-3 (in eng).

60.   Wentworth P, Jr., *et al.* (2002) Evidence for antibody-catalyzed ozone formation in bacterial killing and inflammation. (Translated from eng) *Science* 298(5601):2195-2199 (in eng).

61. Gronwall C, Vas J, & Silverman GJ (2012) Protective Roles of Natural IgM Antibodies. (Translated from eng) *Front Immunol* 3:66 (in eng).

62. Lutz HU & Miescher S (2008) Natural antibodies in health and disease: an overview of the first international workshop on natural antibodies in health and disease. (Translated from eng) *Autoimmun Rev* 7(6):405-409 (in eng).

63. Chou MY, *et al.* (2009) Oxidation-specific epitopes are dominant targets of innate natural antibodies in mice and humans. (Translated from eng) *J Clin Invest* 119(5):1335-1349 (in eng).

64. Binder CJ, *et al.* (2003) Pneumococcal vaccination decreases atherosclerotic lesion formation: molecular mimicry between Streptococcus pneumoniae and oxidized LDL. (Translated from eng) *Nat Med* 9(6):736-743 (in eng).

65. Chen Y, Park YB, Patel E, & Silverman GJ (2009) IgM antibodies to apoptosis-associated determinants recruit C1q and enhance dendritic cell phagocytosis of apoptotic cells. (Translated from eng) *J Immunol* 182(10):6031-6043 (in eng).

66. Stancliffe RA, Thorpe T, & Zemel MB (2011) Dairy attentuates oxidative and inflammatory stress in metabolic syndrome. (Translated from eng) *Am J Clin Nutr* 94(2):422-430 (in eng).

67. Del Rio D, Stewart AJ, & Pellegrini N (2005) A review of recent studies on malondialdehyde as toxic molecule and biological marker of oxidative stress. (Translated from eng) *Nutr Metab Cardiovasc Dis* 15(4):316-328 (in eng).

68. Kulik L, *et al.* (2009) Pathogenic natural antibodies recognizing annexin IV are required to develop intestinal ischemia-reperfusion injury. (Translated from eng) *J Immunol* 182(9):5363-5373 (in eng).

69. Hardy RR & Hayakawa K (2005) Development of B cells producing natural autoantibodies to thymocytes and senescent erythrocytes. (Translated from eng) *Springer Semin Immunopathol* 26(4):363-375 (in eng).

70. Vollmers HP & Brandlein S (2007) Natural antibodies and cancer. (Translated from eng) *J Autoimmun* 29(4):295-302 (in eng).

71. Fishelson Z, Donin N, Zell S, Schultz S, & Kirschfink M (2003) Obstacles to cancer immunotherapy: expression of membrane complement regulatory proteins (mCRPs) in tumors. (Translated from eng) *Mol Immunol* 40(2-4):109-123 (in eng).

72. Schwartz-Albiez R, Laban S, Eichmuller S, & Kirschfink M (2008) Cytotoxic natural antibodies against human tumours: an option for anti-cancer immunotherapy? (Translated from eng) *Autoimmun Rev* 7(6):491-495 (in eng).

73. Ni M & Lee AS (2007) ER chaperones in mammalian development and human diseases. (Translated from eng) *FEBS Lett* 581(19):3641-3651 (in eng).

74. Cabanes D, *et al.* (2005) Gp96 is a receptor for a novel Listeria monocytogenes virulence factor, Vip, a surface protein. (Translated from eng) *Embo J* 24(15):2827-2838 (in eng).

75. Misra UK, Gonzalez-Gronow M, Gawdi G, Wang F, & Pizzo SV (2004) A novel receptor function for the heat shock protein Grp78: silencing of Grp78 gene expression attenuates alpha2M*-induced signalling. (Translated from eng) *Cell Signal* 16(8):929-938 (in eng).

76. Brandlein S, *et al.* (2003) Natural IgM antibodies and immuno-surveillance mechanisms against epithelial cancer cells in humans. (Translated from eng) *Cancer Res* 63(22):7995-8005 (in eng).

77. Hensel F, *et al.* (1999) Characterization of glycosylphosphatidylino-sitol-linked molecule CD55/decay-accelerating factor as the receptor for antibody SC-1-induced apoptosis. (Translated from eng) *Cancer Res* 59(20):5299-5306 (in eng).

78. Vollmers HP, Dammrich J, Ribbert H, Wozniak E, & Muller-Hermelink HK (1995) Apoptosis of stomach carcinoma cells induced by a human monoclonal antibody. (Translated from eng) *Cancer* 76(4):550-558 (in eng).

79. Vollmers HP, O'Connor R, Muller J, Kirchner T, & Muller-Hermelink HK (1989) SC-1, a functional human monoclonal antibody against autologous stomach carcinoma cells. (Translated from eng) *Cancer Res* 49(9):2471-2476 (in eng).

80. Vollmers HP, *et al.* (1998) Adjuvant therapy for gastric adeno-carcinoma with the apoptosis-inducing human monoclonal antibody SC-1: first clinical and histopathological results. (Translated from eng) *Oncol Rep* 5(3):549-552 (in eng).

81. Vollmers HP, *et al.* (1998) Tumor-specific apoptosis induced by the human monoclonal antibody SC-1: a new therapeutical approach for stomach cancer. (Translated from eng) *Oncol Rep* 5(1):35-40 (in eng).

82. Casali P & Notkins AL (1989) CD5+ B lymphocytes, polyreactive antibodies and the human B-cell repertoire. (Translated from eng) *Immunol Today* 10(11):364-368 (in eng).

83. Yednock TA, *et al.* (1992) Prevention of experimental autoimmune encephalomyelitis by antibodies against alpha 4 beta 1 integrin. (Translated from eng) *Nature* 356(6364):63-66 (in eng).

84. Polman CH, *et al.* (2006) A randomized, placebo-controlled trial of natalizumab for relapsing multiple sclerosis. (Translated from eng) *N Engl J Med* 354(9):899-910 (in eng).

85. Rudick RA, *et al.* (2006) Natalizumab plus interferon beta-1a for relapsing multiple sclerosis. (Translated from eng) *N Engl J Med* 354(9):911-923 (in eng).

86. Bloomgren G, *et al.* (2012) Risk of natalizumab-associated progressive multifocal leukoencephalopathy. (Translated from eng) *N Engl J Med* 366(20):1870-1880 (in eng).

87. Coles AJ, *et al.* (2012) Alemtuzumab for patients with relapsing multiple sclerosis after disease-modifying therapy: a randomised controlled phase 3 trial. (Translated from eng) *Lancet* 380(9856):1829-1839 (in eng).

88. Hauser SL, *et al.* (2008) B-cell depletion with rituximab in relapsing-remitting multiple sclerosis. (Translated from eng) *N Engl J Med* 358(7):676-688 (in eng).

89. Hawker K, *et al.* (2009) Rituximab in patients with primary progressive multiple sclerosis: results of a randomized double-blind placebo-controlled multicenter trial. (Translated from eng) *Ann Neurol* 66(4):460-471 (in eng).

90.   Gea-Banacloche JC (2010) Rituximab-associated infections. (Translated from eng) *Seminars in hematology* 47(2):187-198 (in eng).

91.   Bielekova B, *et al.* (2004) Humanized anti-CD25 (daclizumab) inhibits disease activity in multiple sclerosis patients failing to respond to interferon beta. (Translated from eng) *Proc Natl Acad Sci U S A* 101(23):8705-8708 (in eng).

92.   Bielekova B, *et al.* (2006) Regulatory CD56(bright) natural killer cells mediate immunomodulatory effects of IL-2Ralpha-targeted therapy (daclizumab) in multiple sclerosis. (Translated from eng) *Proc Natl Acad Sci U S A* 103(15):5941-5946 (in eng).

93.   Kappos L, *et al.* (2011) Ocrelizumab in relapsing-remitting multiple sclerosis: a phase 2, randomised, placebo-controlled, multicentre trial. (Translated from eng) *Lancet* 378(9805):1779-1787 (in eng).

94.   Hutas G (2008) Ocrelizumab, a humanized monoclonal antibody against CD20 for inflammatory disorders and B-cell malignancies. (Translated from eng) *Curr Opin Investig Drugs* 9(11):1206-1215 (in eng).

95.   Sorensen PS, *et al.* (2014) Safety and efficacy of ofatumumab in relapsing-remitting multiple sclerosis: a phase 2 study. (Translated from eng) *Neurology* 82(7):573-581 (in eng).

96.   Lacroix-Desmazes S, Mouthon L, Coutinho A, & Kazatchkine MD (1995) Analysis of the natural human IgG antibody repertoire: life-long stability of reactivities towards self antigens contrasts with age-dependent diversification of reactivities against bacterial antigens. (Translated from eng) *Eur J Immunol* 25(9):2598-2604 (in eng).

97.   Mouthon L, *et al.* (1995) Analysis of the normal human IgG antibody repertoire. Evidence that IgG autoantibodies of healthy adults recognize a limited and conserved set of protein antigens in homologous tissues. (Translated from eng) *J Immunol* 154(11):5769-5778 (in eng).

98.   Nobrega A, *et al.* (1993) Global analysis of antibody repertoires. II. Evidence for specificity, self-selection and the immunological "homunculus" of antibodies in normal serum. (Translated from eng) *Eur J Immunol* 23(11):2851-2859 (in eng).

99.   Varela F, *et al.* (1991) Population dynamics of natural antibodies in normal and autoimmune individuals. (Translated from eng) *Proc Natl Acad Sci U S A* 88(13):5917-5921 (in eng).

100. Varela FJ & Coutinho A (1991) Second generation immune networks. (Translated from eng) *Immunol Today* 12(5):159-166 (in eng).

101. Gelfand EW (2006) Differences between IGIV products: impact on clinical outcome. (Translated from eng) *Int Immunopharmacol* 6(4):592-599 (in eng).

102. Bayry J, Negi VS, & Kaveri SV (2011) Intravenous immunoglobulin therapy in rheumatic diseases. (Translated from eng) *Nat Rev Rheumatol* 7(6):349-359 (in eng).

103. Blasczyk R, Westhoff U, & Grosse-Wilde H (1993) Soluble CD4, CD8, and HLA molecules in commercial immunoglobulin preparations. (Translated from eng) *Lancet* 341(8848):789-790 (in eng).

104. Lam L, Whitsett CF, McNicholl JM, Hodge TW, & Hooper J (1993) Immunologically active proteins in intravenous immunoglobulin. (Translated from eng) *Lancet* 342(8872):678 (in eng).

105. Buchacher A & Iberer G (2006) Purification of intravenous immunoglobulin G from human plasma--aspects of yield and virus safety. (Translated from eng) *Biotechnol J* 1(2):148-163 (in eng).

106. Imbach P, *et al.* (1981) High-dose intravenous gammaglobulin for idiopathic thrombocytopenic purpura in childhood. (Translated from eng) *Lancet* 1(8232):1228-1231 (in eng).

107. Fehr J, Hofmann V, & Kappeler U (1982) Transient reversal of thrombocytopenia in idiopathic thrombocytopenic purpura by high-dose intravenous gamma globulin. (Translated from eng) *N Engl J Med* 306(21):1254-1258 (in eng).

108. Notarangelo LD (2010) Primary immunodeficiencies. (Translated from eng) *J Allergy Clin Immunol* 125(2 Suppl 2):S182-194 (in eng).

109. Kazatchkine MD & Kaveri SV (2001) Immunomodulation of autoimmune and inflammatory diseases with intravenous immune globulin. (Translated from eng) *N Engl J Med* 345(10):747-755 (in eng).

110. Orange JS, *et al.* (2006) Use of intravenous immunoglobulin in human disease: a review of evidence by members of the Primary Immunodeficiency Committee of the American Academy of Allergy, Asthma and Immunology. (Translated from eng) *J Allergy Clin Immunol* 117(4 Suppl):S525-553 (in eng).

111. Tha-In T, Bayry J, Metselaar HJ, Kaveri SV, & Kwekkeboom J (2008) Modulation of the cellular immune system by intravenous immunoglobulin. (Translated from eng) *Trends Immunol* 29(12):608-615 (in eng).

112. Casadei DH, *et al.* (2001) A randomized and prospective study comparing treatment with high-dose intravenous immunoglobulin with monoclonal antibodies for rescue of kidney grafts with steroid-resistant rejection. (Translated from eng) *Transplantation* 71(1):53-58 (in eng).

113. Luke PP, *et al.* (2001) Reversal of steroid- and anti-lymphocyte antibody-resistant rejection using intravenous immunoglobulin (IVIG) in renal transplant recipients. (Translated from eng) *Transplantation* 72(3):419-422 (in eng).

114. Sokos DR, Berger M, & Lazarus HM (2002) Intravenous immunoglobulin: appropriate indications and uses in hematopoietic stem cell transplantation. (Translated from eng) *Biol Blood Marrow Transplant* 8(3):117-130 (in eng).

115. Buttmann M, Kaveri S, & Hartung HP (2013) Polyclonal immunoglobulin G for autoimmune demyelinating nervous system disorders. (Translated from eng) *Trends Pharmacol Sci* 34(8):445-457 (in eng).

116. Fazekas F, Deisenhammer F, Strasser-Fuchs S, Nahler G, & Mamoli B (1997) Randomised placebo-controlled trial of monthly intravenous immunoglobulin therapy in relapsing-remitting multiple sclerosis. Austrian Immunoglobulin in Multiple Sclerosis Study Group. (Translated from eng) *Lancet* 349(9052):589-593 (in eng).

117. Sorensen PS, *et al.* (1998) Intravenous immunoglobulin G reduces MRI activity in relapsing multiple sclerosis. (Translated from eng) *Neurology* 50(5):1273-1281 (in eng).

118. Lewanska M, Siger-Zajdel M, & Selmaj K (2002) No difference in efficacy of two different doses of intravenous immunoglobulins in MS: clinical and MRI assessment. (Translated from eng) *Eur J Neurol* 9(6):565-572 (in eng).

119. Haas J, Maas-Enriquez M, & Hartung HP (2005) Intravenous immunoglobulins in the treatment of relapsing remitting multiple sclerosis--results of a retrospective multicenter observational study over five years. (Translated from eng) *Mult Scler* 11(5):562-567 (in eng).

120. Noseworthy JH, *et al.* (2000) IV immunoglobulin does not reverse established weakness in MS. (Translated from eng) *Neurology* 55(8):1135-1143 (in eng).

121. Fazekas F, *et al.* (2008) Intravenous immunoglobulin in relapsing-remitting multiple sclerosis: a dose-finding trial. (Translated from eng) *Neurology* 71(4):265-271 (in eng).

122. Bayry J, Hartung HP, & Kaveri SV (2015) IVIg for relapsing-remitting multiple sclerosis: promises and uncertainties. (Translated from Eng) *Trends Pharmacol Sci* (in Eng).

123. Nicholas R & Chataway J (2009) Multiple sclerosis. (Translated from eng) *BMJ Clin Evid* 2009 (in eng).

124. Rieben R, *et al.* (1999) Immunoglobulin M-enriched human intravenous immunoglobulin prevents complement activation in vitro and in vivo in a rat model of acute inflammation. (Translated from eng) *Blood* 93(3):942-951 (in eng).

125. Walpen AJ, Laumonier T, Aebi C, Mohacsi PJ, & Rieben R (2004) Immunoglobulin M-enriched intravenous immunoglobulin inhibits classical pathway complement activation, but not bactericidal activity of human serum. (Translated from eng) *Xenotransplantation* 11(2):141-148 (in eng).

126. Stehr SN, *et al.* (2008) Effects of IGM-enriched solution on polymorphonuclear neutrophil function, bacterial clearance, and lung histology in endotoxemia. (Translated from eng) *Shock* 29(2):167-172 (in eng).

127. Hurez V, *et al.* (1997) Pooled normal human polyspecific IgM contains neutralizing anti-idiotypes to IgG autoantibodies of autoimmune patients and protects from experimental autoimmune disease. (Translated from eng) *Blood* 90(10):4004-4013 (in eng).

128. Varambally S, *et al.* (2004) Natural human polyreactive IgM induce apoptosis of lymphoid cell lines and human peripheral blood mononuclear cells. (Translated from eng) *Int Immunol* 16(3):517-524 (in eng).

129. Vassilev T, *et al.* (2006) IgM-enriched human intravenous immuno-globulin suppresses T lymphocyte functions in vitro and delays the activation of T lymphocytes in hu-SCID mice. (Translated from eng) *Clin Exp Immunol* 145(1):108-115 (in eng).

130. Acorda Therapeutics Inc (2015) An Intravenous Infusion Study of rHIgM22 in Patients With Multiple Sclerosis. Clinical Trials Identifier - NCT01803867 | Weblink - http://1.usa.gov/1N2gsHJ.

131. Greenberg BM, *et al.* (2015) Safety and Tolerability of the Re-myelinating Therapeutic Antibody rHIgM22 in Patients with Stable Multiple Sclerosis. in *Poster N° - P4.339 | ACO P5130, 67th AAN Annual Meeting | American Academy of Neurology® April 18-25, Washington, DC, USA* (Washington, DC, USA).

132. Wittenberg NJ, *et al.* (2012) High-affinity binding of remyelinating natural autoantibodies to myelin-mimicking lipid bilayers revealed by nanohole surface plasmon resonance. (Translated from eng) *Anal Chem* 84(14):6031-6039 (in eng).

133. Paz Soldan MM, *et al.* (2003) Remyelination-promoting antibodies activate distinct Ca2+ influx pathways in astrocytes and oligo-dendrocytes: relationship to the mechanism of myelin repair. (Translated from eng) *Mol Cell Neurosci* 22(1):14-24 (in eng).

134. Eisenbarth GS, Walsh FS, & Nirenberg M (1979) Monoclonal antibody to a plasma membrane antigen of neurons. *Proc Natl Acad Sci U S A* 76(10):4913-4917.

135. Burger D, Perruisseau G, Simon M, & Steck AJ (1992) Comparison of the N-linked oligosaccharide structures of the two major human myelin glycoproteins MAG and P0: assessment of the structures

bearing the epitope for HNK-1 and human monoclonal immuno-globulin M found in demyelinating neuropathy. (Translated from eng) *J Neurochem* 58(3):854-861 (in eng).

136. Burger D, Simon M, Perruisseau G, & Steck AJ (1990) The epitope(s) recognized by HNK-1 antibody and IgM paraprotein in neuropathy is present on several N-linked oligosaccharide structures on human P0 and myelin-associated glycoprotein. (Translated from eng) *J Neurochem* 54(5):1569-1575 (in eng).

137. Schachner M (1982) Cell type-specific surface antigens in the mammalian nervous system. (Translated from eng) *J Neurochem* 39(1):1-8 (in eng).

138. Inoko E, *et al.* (2010) Developmental stage-dependent expression of an alpha2,8-trisialic acid unit on glycoproteins in mouse brain. (Translated from eng) *Glycobiology* 20(7):916-928 (in eng).

139. Dubois C, *et al.* (1986) Monoclonal antibody 18B8, which detects synapse-associated antigens, binds to ganglioside GT3 (II3 (NeuAc)3LacCer). (Translated from eng) *J Biol Chem* 261(8):3826-3830 (in eng).

140. Heffer-Lauc M, Cacic M, & Serman D (1998) C-series polysialogangliosides are expressed on stellate neurons of adult human cerebellum. (Translated from eng) *Glycoconj J* 15(4):423-426 (in eng).

141. Asakura K, Miller DJ, Pease LR, & Rodriguez M (1998) Targeting of IgMkappa antibodies to oligodendrocytes promotes CNS remye-lination. (Translated from eng) *J Neurosci* 18(19):7700-7708 (in eng).

142. Kirschning E, *et al.* (1999) Primary structure of the antigen-binding domains of a human oligodendrocyte-reactive IgM monoclonal antibody derived from a patient with multiple sclerosis. (Translated from eng) *J Neuroimmunol* 99(1):122-130 (in eng).

143. Sommer I & Schachner M (1981) Monoclonal antibodies (O1 to O4) to oligodendrocyte cell surfaces: an immunocytological study in the central nervous system. (Translated from eng) *Dev Biol* 83(2):311-327 (in eng).

144. Willison HJ & Yuki N (2002) Peripheral neuropathies and anti-glycolipid antibodies. (Translated from eng) *Brain* 125(Pt 12):2591-2625 (in eng).

145. Carpo M, *et al.* (2000) Anti-sulfatide IgM antibodies in peripheral neuropathy. (Translated from eng) *Journal of the neurological sciences* 176(2):144-150 (in eng).

146. Ledeen RW (1984) Biology of gangliosides: neuritogenic and neuro-notrophic properties. (Translated from eng) *J Neurosci Res* 12(2-3):147-159 (in eng).

147. Bradley WG, *et al.* (1988) Double-blind controlled trials of Cronassial in chronic neuromuscular diseases and ataxia. (Translated from eng) *Neurology* 38(11):1731-1739 (in eng).

148. Ponzin D, *et al.* (1991) Effects of gangliosides on the expression of autoimmune demyelination in the peripheral nervous system. (Translated from eng) *Ann Neurol* 30(5):678-685 (in eng).

149. Ilyas AA & Chen ZW (2007) Lewis rats immunized with GM1 ganglioside do not develop peripheral neuropathy. (Translated from eng) *J Neuroimmunol* 188(1-2):34-38 (in eng).

150. Yuki N, *et al.* (2004) Carbohydrate mimicry between human ganglioside GM1 and Campylobacter jejuni lipooligosaccharide causes Guillain-Barre syndrome. (Translated from eng) *Proc Natl Acad Sci U S A* 101(31):11404-11409 (in eng).

151. Kaida K & Kusunoki S (2013) [Immune-mediated neuropathy and anti-glycolipid antibodies]. (Translated from jpn) *Brain and nerve = Shinkei kenkyu no shinpo* 65(4):413-423 (in jpn).

152. Rojas-Garcia R, Gallardo E, & Illa I (2013) Paraproteinemic neuropathies. (Translated from eng) *Presse medicale* 42(6 Pt 2):e225-234 (in eng).

153. Dyck PJ, *et al.* (1991) Plasma exchange in polyneuropathy associated with monoclonal gammopathy of undetermined significance. (Translated from eng) *N Engl J Med* 325(21):1482-1486 (in eng).

154. Nobile-Orazio E, Meucci N, Baldini L, Di Troia A, & Scarlato G (2000) Long-term prognosis of neuropathy associated with anti-

MAG IgM M-proteins and its relationship to immune therapies. (Translated from eng) *Brain* 123 (Pt 4):710-717 (in eng).

155. Mygland A & Monstad P (2003) Chronic acquired demyelinating symmetric polyneuropathy classified by pattern of weakness. (Translated from eng) *Arch Neurol* 60(2):260-264 (in eng).

156. Thies WBL (2013) Alzheimer's Association: 2013 Alzheimers disease facts and figures. *Alzheimers Dement* 9:208-245.

157. Mattson MP (2004) Pathways towards and away from Alzheimer's disease. (Translated from eng) *Nature* 430(7000):631-639 (in eng).

158. Reddy PH, *et al.* (2010) Amyloid-beta and mitochondria in aging and Alzheimer's disease: implications for synaptic damage and cognitive decline. (Translated from eng) *J Alzheimers Dis* 20 Suppl 2:S499-512 (in eng).

159. Selkoe DJ (2001) Alzheimer's disease: genes, proteins, and therapy. (Translated from eng) *Physiol Rev* 81(2):741-766 (in eng).

160. Janus C, *et al.* (2000) A beta peptide immunization reduces behavioural impairment and plaques in a model of Alzheimer's disease. (Translated from eng) *Nature* 408(6815):979-982 (in eng).

161. Morgan D, *et al.* (2000) A beta peptide vaccination prevents memory loss in an animal model of Alzheimer's disease. (Translated from eng) *Nature* 408(6815):982-985 (in eng).

162. Bard F, *et al.* (2000) Peripherally administered antibodies against amyloid beta-peptide enter the central nervous system and reduce pathology in a mouse model of Alzheimer disease. (Translated from eng) *Nat Med* 6(8):916-919 (in eng).

163. DeMattos RB, *et al.* (2001) Peripheral anti-A beta antibody alters CNS and plasma A beta clearance and decreases brain A beta burden in a mouse model of Alzheimer's disease. (Translated from eng) *Proc Natl Acad Sci U S A* 98(15):8850-8855 (in eng).

164. Dodart JC, *et al.* (2002) Immunization reverses memory deficits without reducing brain Abeta burden in Alzheimer's disease model. (Translated from eng) *Nature neuroscience* 5(5):452-457 (in eng).

165. Walsh DM & Selkoe DJ (2004) Deciphering the molecular basis of memory failure in Alzheimer's disease. (Translated from eng) *Neuron* 44(1):181-193 (in eng).

166. Schenk D, *et al.* (1999) Immunization with amyloid-beta attenuates Alzheimer-disease-like pathology in the PDAPP mouse. (Translated from eng) *Nature* 400(6740):173-177 (in eng).

167. Bacskai BJ, *et al.* (2002) Non-Fc-mediated mechanisms are involved in clearance of amyloid-beta in vivo by immunotherapy. (Translated from eng) *J Neurosci* 22(18):7873-7878 (in eng).

168. Morgan D (2006) Immunotherapy for Alzheimer's disease. (Translated from eng) *J Alzheimers Dis* 9(3 Suppl):425-432 (in eng).

169. Gilman S, *et al.* (2005) Clinical effects of Abeta immunization (AN1792) in patients with AD in an interrupted trial. (Translated from eng) *Neurology* 64(9):1553-1562 (in eng).

170. Holmes C, *et al.* (2008) Long-term effects of Abeta42 immunisation in Alzheimer's disease: follow-up of a randomised, placebo-controlled phase I trial. (Translated from eng) *Lancet* 372(9634):216-223 (in eng).

171. Boche D, *et al.* (2010) Reduction of aggregated Tau in neuronal processes but not in the cell bodies after Abeta42 immunisation in Alzheimer's disease. (Translated from eng) *Acta Neuropathol* 120(1):13-20 (in eng).

172. Serrano-Pozo A, *et al.* (2010) Beneficial effect of human anti-amyloid-beta active immunization on neurite morphology and tau pathology. (Translated from eng) *Brain* 133(Pt 5):1312-1327 (in eng).

173. Lemere CA & Masliah E (2010) Can Alzheimer disease be prevented by amyloid-beta immunotherapy? (Translated from eng) *Nat Rev Neurol* 6(2):108-119 (in eng).

174. Farlow MR, *et al.* (2015) Long-term treatment with active Abeta immunotherapy with CAD106 in mild Alzheimer's disease. (Translated from eng) *Alzheimers Res Ther* 7(1):23 (in eng).

175. Schneeberger A, *et al.* (2009) Development of AFFITOPE vaccines for Alzheimer's disease (AD)--from concept to clinical testing. (Translated from eng) *J Nutr Health Aging* 13(3):264-267 (in eng).

176. Orgogozo JM, *et al.* (2003) Subacute meningoencephalitis in a subset of patients with AD after Abeta42 immunization. (Translated from eng) *Neurology* 61(1):46-54 (in eng).

177. Blennow K, *et al.* (2012) Effect of immunotherapy with bapineuzumab on cerebrospinal fluid biomarker levels in patients with mild to moderate Alzheimer disease. (Translated from eng) *Arch Neurol* 69(8):1002-1010 (in eng).

178. Doody RS, *et al.* (2014) Phase 3 trials of solanezumab for mild-to-moderate Alzheimer's disease. (Translated from eng) *N Engl J Med* 370(4):311-321 (in eng).

179. Burstein AH, *et al.* (2013) Safety and pharmacology of ponezumab (PF-04360365) after a single 10-minute intravenous infusion in subjects with mild to moderate Alzheimer disease. (Translated from eng) *Clinical neuropharmacology* 36(1):8-13 (in eng).

180. Fillit H, Hess G, Hill J, Bonnet P, & Toso C (2009) IV immunoglobulin is associated with a reduced risk of Alzheimer disease and related disorders. (Translated from eng) *Neurology* 73(3):180-185 (in eng).

181. Dodel RC, *et al.* (2004) Intravenous immunoglobulins containing antibodies against beta-amyloid for the treatment of Alzheimer's disease. (Translated from eng) *J Neurol Neurosurg Psychiatry* 75(10):1472-1474 (in eng).

182. Relkin NR, *et al.* (2009) 18-Month study of intravenous immunoglobulin for treatment of mild Alzheimer disease. (Translated from eng) *Neurobiol Aging* 30(11):1728-1736 (in eng).

183. Dodel R, *et al.* (2013) Intravenous immunoglobulin for treatment of mild-to-moderate Alzheimer's disease: a phase 2, randomised, double-blind, placebo-controlled, dose-finding trial. (Translated from eng) *Lancet Neurol* 12(3):233-243 (in eng).

184. Loeffler DA (2013) Intravenous immunoglobulin and Alzheimer's disease: what now? (Translated from eng) *J Neuroinflammation* 10:70 (in eng).

185. Dodel R, *et al.* (2002) Human antibodies against amyloid beta peptide: a potential treatment for Alzheimer's disease. (Translated from eng) *Ann Neurol* 52(2):253-256 (in eng).

186. Balakrishnan K, Andrei-Selmer LC, Selmer T, Bacher M, & Dodel R (2010) Comparison of intravenous immunoglobulins for naturally occurring autoantibodies against amyloid-beta. (Translated from eng) *J Alzheimers Dis* 20(1):135-143 (in eng).

187. Klaver AC, Finke JM, Digambaranath J, Balasubramaniam M, & Loeffler DA (2010) Antibody concentrations to Abeta1-42 monomer and soluble oligomers in untreated and antibody-antigen-dissociated intravenous immunoglobulin preparations. (Translated from eng) *Int Immunopharmacol* 10(1):115-119 (in eng).

188. Smith LM, Coffey MP, Klaver AC, & Loeffler DA (2013) Intravenous immunoglobulin products contain specific antibodies to recombinant human tau protein. (Translated from eng) *Int Immunopharmacol* 16(4):424-428 (in eng).

189. Du Y, *et al.* (2001) Reduced levels of amyloid beta-peptide antibody in Alzheimer disease. (Translated from eng) *Neurology* 57(5):801-805 (in eng).

190. Weksler ME, *et al.* (2002) Patients with Alzheimer disease have lower levels of serum anti-amyloid peptide antibodies than healthy elderly individuals. (Translated from eng) *Experimental gerontology* 37(7):943-948 (in eng).

191. Szabo P, Relkin N, & Weksler ME (2008) Natural human antibodies to amyloid beta peptide. (Translated from eng) *Autoimmun Rev* 7(6):415-420 (in eng).

192. Sigurdsson EM, *et al.* (2004) An attenuated immune response is sufficient to enhance cognition in an Alzheimer's disease mouse model immunized with amyloid-beta derivatives. (Translated from eng) *J Neurosci* 24(28):6277-6282 (in eng).

193. Britschgi M, *et al.* (2009) Neuroprotective natural antibodies to assemblies of amyloidogenic peptides decrease with normal aging and advancing Alzheimer's disease. (Translated from eng) *Proc Natl Acad Sci U S A* 106(29):12145-12150 (in eng).

194. Mengel D, *et al.* (2013) Naturally occurring autoantibodies interfere with beta-amyloid metabolism and improve cognition in a transgenic mouse model of Alzheimer's disease 24 h after single treatment. (Translated from eng) *Transl Psychiatry* 3:e236 (in eng).

195. Moreth J, Mavoungou C, & Schindowski K (2013) Passive anti-amyloid immunotherapy in Alzheimer's disease: What are the most promising targets? (Translated from eng) *Immun Ageing* 10(1):18 (in eng).

196. McLaurin J, *et al.* (2002) Therapeutically effective antibodies against amyloid-beta peptide target amyloid-beta residues 4-10 and inhibit cytotoxicity and fibrillogenesis. (Translated from eng) *Nat Med* 8(11):1263-1269 (in eng).

197. Taguchi H, *et al.* (2008) Autoantibody-catalyzed hydrolysis of amyloid beta peptide. (Translated from eng) *J Biol Chem* 283(8):4714-4722 (in eng).

198. Nishiyama Y, *et al.* (2014) Metal-dependent amyloid beta-degrading catalytic antibody construct. (Translated from eng) *Journal of biotechnology* 180:17-22 (in eng).

199. Hammel P, *et al.* (1990) Acute hepatitis after tetrahydroaminoacridine administration for Alzheimer's disease. (Translated from eng) *J Clin Gastroenterol* 12(3):329-331 (in eng).

200. Becker RE & Greig NH (2012) Increasing the success rate for Alzheimer's disease drug discovery and development. (Translated from eng) *Expert Opin Drug Discov* 7(4):367-370 (in eng).

201. Cummings J (2010) What can be inferred from the interruption of the semagacestat trial for treatment of Alzheimer's disease? (Translated from eng) *Biol Psychiatry* 68(10):876-878 (in eng).

202. Cummings JL, Morstorf T, & Zhong K (2014) Alzheimer's disease drug-development pipeline: few candidates, frequent failures. (Translated from eng) *Alzheimers Res Ther* 6(4):37 (in eng).

203. Mullane K & Williams M (2013) Alzheimer's therapeutics: continued clinical failures question the validity of the amyloid hypothesis-but

what lies beyond? (Translated from eng) *Biochem Pharmacol* 85(3):289-305 (in eng).

204. Geerts H (2009) Of mice and men: bridging the translational disconnect in CNS drug discovery. (Translated from eng) *CNS Drugs* 23(11):915-926 (in eng).

205. Li C, Ebrahimi A, & Schluesener H (2013) Drug pipeline in neurodegeneration based on transgenic mice models of Alzheimer's disease. (Translated from eng) *Ageing Res Rev* 12(1):116-140 (in eng).

206. Wilcock DM (2010) The usefulness and challenges of transgenic mouse models in the study of Alzheimer's disease. (Translated from eng) *CNS Neurol Disord Drug Targets* 9(4):386-394 (in eng).

207. Jaturapatporn D, Isaac MG, McCleery J, & Tabet N (2012) Aspirin, steroidal and non-steroidal anti-inflammatory drugs for the treatment of Alzheimer's disease. (Translated from eng) *Cochrane Database Syst Rev* 2:CD006378 (in eng).

208. Michaelis ML, Georg G, Telikepalli H, McIntosh M, & Rajewski RA (2006) Ongoing in vivo studies with cytoskeletal drugs in tau transgenic mice. (Translated from eng) *Curr Alzheimer Res* 3(3):215-219 (in eng).

209. Sherrington R, *et al.* (1995) Cloning of a gene bearing missense mutations in early-onset familial Alzheimer's disease. (Translated from eng) *Nature* 375(6534):754-760 (in eng).

210. McKeith IG, *et al.* (2000) Prospective validation of consensus criteria for the diagnosis of dementia with Lewy bodies. (Translated from eng) *Neurology* 54(5):1050-1058 (in eng).

211. McKeith IG, *et al.* (1996) Consensus guidelines for the clinical and pathologic diagnosis of dementia with Lewy bodies (DLB): report of the consortium on DLB international workshop. (Translated from eng) *Neurology* 47(5):1113-1124 (in eng).

212. Mahowald MW, Bornemann MA, & Schenck CH (2010) When and where do synucleinopathies begin? (Translated from eng) *Neurology* 75(6):488-489 (in eng).

213. Galasko D, *et al.* (1994) Clinical-neuropathological correlations in Alzheimer's disease and related dementias. (Translated from eng) *Arch Neurol* 51(9):888-895 (in eng).

214. Schulz-Schaeffer WJ (2010) The synaptic pathology of alpha-synuclein aggregation in dementia with Lewy bodies, Parkinson's disease and Parkinson's disease dementia. (Translated from eng) *Acta Neuropathol* 120(2):131-143 (in eng).

215. Spillantini MG & Goedert M (2000) The alpha-synucleinopathies: Parkinson's disease, dementia with Lewy bodies, and multiple system atrophy. (Translated from eng) *Ann N Y Acad Sci* 920:16-27 (in eng).

216. Spillantini MG, *et al.* (1997) Alpha-synuclein in Lewy bodies. (Translated from eng) *Nature* 388(6645):839-840 (in eng).

217. Wakabayashi K, Matsumoto K, Takayama K, Yoshimoto M, & Takahashi H (1997) NACP, a presynaptic protein, immunoreactivity in Lewy bodies in Parkinson's disease. (Translated from eng) *Neurosci Lett* 239(1):45-48 (in eng).

218. Kruger R, *et al.* (1998) Ala30Pro mutation in the gene encoding alpha-synuclein in Parkinson's disease. (Translated from eng) *Nat Genet* 18(2):106-108 (in eng).

219. Polymeropoulos MH, *et al.* (1997) Mutation in the alpha-synuclein gene identified in families with Parkinson's disease. (Translated from eng) *Science* 276(5321):2045-2047 (in eng).

220. Masliah E, *et al.* (2000) Dopaminergic loss and inclusion body formation in alpha-synuclein mice: implications for neurodegenerative disorders. (Translated from eng) *Science* 287(5456):1265-1269 (in eng).

221. Conway KA, *et al.* (2000) Acceleration of oligomerization, not fibrillization, is a shared property of both alpha-synuclein mutations linked to early-onset Parkinson's disease: implications for pathogenesis and therapy. (Translated from eng) *Proc Natl Acad Sci U S A* 97(2):571-576 (in eng).

222. Volles MJ & Lansbury PT, Jr. (2003) Zeroing in on the pathogenic form of alpha-synuclein and its mechanism of neurotoxicity in Parkinson's disease. (Translated from eng) *Biochemistry* 42(26):7871-7878 (in eng).

223. Desplats P, *et al.* (2009) Inclusion formation and neuronal cell death through neuron-to-neuron transmission of alpha-synuclein. (Translated from eng) *Proc Natl Acad Sci U S A* 106(31):13010-13015 (in eng).

224. Masliah E, *et al.* (2011) Passive immunization reduces behavioral and neuropathological deficits in an alpha-synuclein transgenic model of Lewy body disease. (Translated from eng) *PLoS One* 6(4):e19338 (in eng).

225. Games D, *et al.* (2013) Axonopathy in an alpha-synuclein transgenic model of Lewy body disease is associated with extensive accumulation of C-terminal-truncated alpha-synuclein. (Translated from eng) *Am J Pathol* 182(3):940-953 (in eng).

226. Games D, *et al.* (2014) Reducing C-terminal-truncated alpha-synuclein by immunotherapy attenuates neurodegeneration and propagation in Parkinson's disease-like models. (Translated from eng) *J Neurosci* 34(28):9441-9454 (in eng).

227. Papachroni KK, *et al.* (2007) Autoantibodies to alpha-synuclein in inherited Parkinson's disease. (Translated from eng) *J Neurochem* 101(3):749-756 (in eng).

228. Neff F, *et al.* (2008) Immunotherapy and naturally occurring autoantibodies in neurodegenerative disorders. (Translated from eng) *Autoimmun Rev* 7(6):501-507 (in eng).

229. Besong-Agbo D, *et al.* (2013) Naturally occurring alpha-synuclein autoantibody levels are lower in patients with Parkinson disease. (Translated from eng) *Neurology* 80(2):169-175 (in eng).

230. Heinzel S, *et al.* (2014) Naturally occurring alpha-synuclein autoantibodies in Parkinson's disease: sources of (error) variance in biomarker assays. (Translated from eng) *PLoS One* 9(12):e114566 (in eng).

231. Deleersnijder A, Gerard M, Debyser Z, & Baekelandt V (2013) The remarkable conformational plasticity of alpha-synuclein: blessing or curse? (Translated from eng) *Trends Mol Med* 19(6):368-377 (in eng).

232. Yanamandra K, *et al.* (2011) alpha-synuclein reactive antibodies as diagnostic biomarkers in blood sera of Parkinson's disease patients. (Translated from eng) *PLoS One* 6(4):e18513 (in eng).

233. Peretz D, *et al.* (2001) Antibodies inhibit prion propagation and clear cell cultures of prion infectivity. (Translated from eng) *Nature* 412(6848):739-743 (in eng).

234. White AR, *et al.* (2003) Monoclonal antibodies inhibit prion replication and delay the development of prion disease. (Translated from eng) *Nature* 422(6927):80-83 (in eng).

235. Heppner FL, *et al.* (2001) Prevention of scrapie pathogenesis by transgenic expression of anti-prion protein antibodies. (Translated from eng) *Science* 294(5540):178-182 (in eng).

236. Sigurdsson EM, *et al.* (2003) Anti-prion antibodies for prophylaxis following prion exposure in mice. (Translated from eng) *Neurosci Lett* 336(3):185-187 (in eng).

237. Solforosi L, *et al.* (2004) Cross-linking cellular prion protein triggers neuronal apoptosis in vivo. (Translated from eng) *Science* 303(5663):1514-1516 (in eng).

238. Bade S & Frey A (2007) Potential of active and passive immunizations for the prevention and therapy of transmissible spongiform encephalopathies. (Translated from eng) *Expert review of vaccines* 6(2):153-168 (in eng).

239. Wei X, *et al.* (2012) Human anti-prion antibodies block prion peptide fibril formation and neurotoxicity. (Translated from eng) *J Biol Chem* 287(16):12858-12866 (in eng).

240. Watzlawik J, *et al.* (2006) Prion protein helix1 promotes aggregation but is not converted into beta-sheet. (Translated from eng) *J Biol Chem* 281(40):30242-30250 (in eng).

241. Broman T (1964) Blood-Brain Barrier Damage in Multiple Sclerosis Supravital Test-Observations. (Translated from eng) *Acta Neurol Scand Suppl* 40:SUPPL 10:21-14 (in eng).

242. McQuaid S, Cunnea P, McMahon J, & Fitzgerald U (2009) The effects of blood-brain barrier disruption on glial cell function in multiple sclerosis. (Translated from eng) *Biochem Soc Trans* 37(Pt 1):329-331 (in eng).

243. Gay D & Esiri M (1991) Blood-brain barrier damage in acute multiple sclerosis plaques. An immunocytological study. (Translated from eng) *Brain* 114 (Pt 1B):557-572 (in eng).

244. Kwon EE & Prineas JW (1994) Blood-brain barrier abnormalities in longstanding multiple sclerosis lesions. An immunohistochemical study. (Translated from eng) *J Neuropathol Exp Neurol* 53(6):625-636 (in eng).

245. Banks WA (2012) Drug delivery to the brain in Alzheimer's disease: consideration of the blood-brain barrier. (Translated from eng) *Advanced drug delivery reviews* 64(7):629-639 (in eng).

246. Banks WA, *et al.* (2002) Passage of amyloid beta protein antibody across the blood-brain barrier in a mouse model of Alzheimer's disease. (Translated from eng) *Peptides* 23(12):2223-2226 (in eng).

247. Bergman I, *et al.* (1998) Pharmacokinetics of IgG and IgM anti-ganglioside antibodies in rats and monkeys after intrathecal administration. (Translated from eng) *The Journal of pharmacology and experimental therapeutics* 284(1):111-115 (in eng).

248. Braen AP, *et al.* (2010) A 4-week intrathecal toxicity and pharmacokinetic study with trastuzumab in cynomolgus monkeys. (Translated from eng) *International journal of toxicology* 29(3):259-267 (in eng).

249. Pepinsky RB, *et al.* (2011) Exposure levels of anti-LINGO-1 Li81 antibody in the central nervous system and dose-efficacy relationships in rat spinal cord remyelination models after systemic administration. (Translated from eng) *The Journal of pharmacology and experimental therapeutics* 339(2):519-529 (in eng).

250. Boado RJ, Lu JZ, Hui EK, Sumbria RK, & Pardridge WM (2013) Pharmacokinetics and brain uptake in the rhesus monkey of a fusion protein of arylsulfatase a and a monoclonal antibody against the human insulin receptor. (Translated from eng) *Biotechnology and bioengineering* 110(5):1456-1465 (in eng).

251. Couch JA, *et al.* (2013) Addressing safety liabilities of TfR bispecific antibodies that cross the blood-brain barrier. (Translated from eng) *Sci Transl Med* 5(183):183ra157, 181-112 (in eng).

252. Spencer BJ & Verma IM (2007) Targeted delivery of proteins across the blood-brain barrier. (Translated from eng) *Proc Natl Acad Sci U S A* 104(18):7594-7599 (in eng).

www.ingramcontent.com/pod-product-compliance
Lightning Source LLC
Chambersburg PA
CBHW061821210326
41599CB00034B/7070